P9-AQF-615

THE FIRE INSIDE

THE FIRE INSIDE

Extinguishing Heartburn and Related Symptoms

M. MICHAEL WOLFE, M.D.
and THOMAS J. NESI

W. W. Norton & Company
New York London

Copyright © 1996 by M. Michael Wolfe, M.D.,
and Thomas J. Nesi

All rights reserved
Printed in the United States of America

First Edition

The text of this book is composed in Imprint 101,
with the display set in Garamond.
Composition and manufacturing by
the Haddon Craftsmen, Inc.
Book design by Chris Welch.

Library of Congress Cataloging-in-Publication Data
Wolfe, M. Michael.
The fire inside : extinguishing heartburn and
related symptoms / M. Michael Wolfe and Thomas J. Nesi.
p. cm.
Includes index.
1. Heartburn. 2. Gastroesophageal reflux. I. Nesi, Thomas J. II.
Title.
RC815.7.W65 1996
616.3'32—dc20   95-10737

ISBN 0-393-03863-7

W. W. Norton & Company, Inc.
500 Fifth Avenue, New York, N.Y. 10110
W. W. Norton & Company Ltd.
10 Coptic Street, London WC1A 1PU

1 2 3 4 5 6 7 8 9 0

This book is dedicated to our parents
and with much love to our wives and children:
Barbara, Jessica, Matt, and Aliza Wolfe
Susan and Chris Nesi

CONTENTS

ACKNOWLEDGMENTS

In our commitment to educate the public about acid reflux disease, we have received invaluable assistance and guidance from a number of superb health care professionals. These include Dr. William Garnett (Richmond, Virginia), Dr. Joel Richter (Cleveland, Ohio), Dr. James Koufman (Winston-Salem, North Carolina), and Dr. Susan Harding (Birmingham, Alabama). We are grateful also to Dr. Michael Parsons, one of the inventors of Tagamet, and Dr. Enar Carlsson, of Hässle Laboratories, each of whom took time to share their wealth of knowledge about drug development. A debt of thanks is due to Dr. James McGuigan and Dr. Phillip Toskes (Gainesville, Florida), who provided outstanding training (to M. M. W.) to gain the expertise necessary for the writing of this book.

We would also like to extend our gratitude to Janet Morse Fox, Barbara Rosenblum-Wolfe, and Susan Jubelirer for their help in the preparation of the manuscript, to Dr. Jerry Trier (Boston, Massachusetts) for his critical evaluation and suggestions, and to Carol Houck Smith of W. W. Norton & Company for her superb editing of the manuscript. Most of all, we thank the many sufferers who spoke with us of their experiences with reflux disease. Their physical and emotional pain led us to address the unfulfilled need of patient education.

M. M. W.

T. J. N.

Introduction

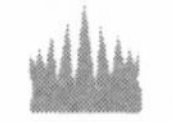

THE MEDICAL REVOLUTION

> Fortune. . . . She either gives a stomach and no food . . . or else a feast / And takes away the stomach.
>
> —*William Shakespeare,* Henry IV, Part II

In the last fifteen years there has been a revolution in the way patients are treated for diseases of the digestive tract. The first part of this revolution made it possible for most people with stomach and duodenal ulcers to live normal, painfree lives without the threat of hospitalization and potentially dangerous surgery.

The second part of this revolution is occurring now, and it is altering the way physicians treat reflux disease and its many associated ailments. The full medical term for acid reflux is "gastroesophageal reflux disease" (GERD). "Gastro" refers to the stomach, and "esophagus" to the part of the body just above the stomach and below the throat. The term "reflux" means "blackflow" and comes from the Latin *re* ("back") and *fluere* ("to flow"). In reflux disease, food mixing with acid flows back *up* the digestive tract sometimes all the way to the mouth, rather than *down* to the intestines. This mixture may cause anything from mild heartburn to lethal lung disease. The reason is that stomach acid is far more powerful than most people realize. It is almost as corrosive as the acid in car batteries that needs to be housed in lead!

Because acid reflux appears in so many disguises, it is sometimes known as the Great Masquerader. Every year sufferers with an odd assortment of debilitating symptoms race from doctor to doctor, clinic to clinic, in the desperate hope of finding relief. With proper diagnosis and treatment, they can find it.

We now understand that many forms of reflux disease must be treated differently to make patients well. But too often this doesn't happen, and suffering continues—on a vast scale. To document this, let's look more closely at acid reflux and its various confusing symptoms.

Heartburn, in one form or another, affects more than one hundred *million* Americans. Sufferers spend an astonishing three *billion* dollars every *year* on medications to treat it. One survey showed that more than twenty-five million Americans take antacids twice a week, and millions more take one or more prescription drugs on a daily basis.

More than twelve million people suffer from asthma, and of those, between one third and two thirds have symptoms or actual underlying illness related to reflux disease. Making matters worse, asthmatics often take medication that *aggravates* acid reflux and, indirectly, the asthma itself. People are amazed to find that such serious lung maladies as pneumonia and chronic bronchitis are also related to acid reflux.

Recent statistics suggest that at least 180,000 people

each year are admitted to emergency rooms with chest pain so severe it is thought to be signaling a heart attack. As with lung conditions, the chest pain is often revealed as reflux disease. Ironically, many patients with chest pain unrelated to heart ailments are dismissed with the diagnosis of anxiety and given medication that only guarantees return visits to the hospital.

As for severe hoarseness, loss of voice, and chronic cough, no truly scientific data are available about their extent (we have estimated a minimum of five million people), but the relationship between these conditions and acid reflux is not undisputed. The volume of people who suffer from reflux disease and throat problems, such as postnasal drip, swells the numbers.

Thus acid reflux and its many medical masquerades can be as incapacitating as they are common, affecting work, family life, education, physical activity, and sleep. Severe reflux disease can be life-threatening and extremely costly.

As a practicing gastroenterologist and specialist in stomach acid-related disorders, I am most disturbed by how much money is wasted—on over-the-counter remedies, outdated prescription drug therapies, or repeated doctor visits—because of the widespread misunderstanding of acid reflux and the inability to recognize and treat it. I commonly see people whose disease has gone unrecognized for years or who *have* been diagnosed but are on remedies that are ineffective or making them worse.

This is the first book written for the general public specifically about acid reflux and its most common related ailments. Its intention is simple: to dispel myths, calm fears, and point sufferers and their families and friends in the direction of the correct diagnostic procedures and therapies, many of which are new. In short, we're going to put people with reflux disease on the path to relief. We'll accomplish this by discussing developments and research that everyone with this painful condition should be aware of:

—How antacids can help you and why sometimes they can *harm* you

—How common over-the-counter and prescription medicines can make your condition worse

—How to tell if your asthma, hoarseness, or chest pain is really reflux disease and what to do about it

—How a recently developed once-a-day prescription drug can stave off surgery, help diagnose your condition, and cure even severe or long-lasting reflux disease

—How a drug combination, developed in Boston at the Brigham and Women's Hospital, can bring you rapid and lasting relief

—Why you may not be taking enough of your present heartburn medication or taking it at the wrong time

—How lifestyle changes (food, exercise, weight loss, even change of clothing) can help and what you can *realistically* accomplish without medicine

—What symptoms, other than heartburn, may indicate serious digestive disease

—How stomach and duodenal ulcers differ from reflux disease and how new therapies promise an end to both

I have also provided a glossary of terms at the end of the book that you may refer to at any time. It is intended to put any complex terms regarding your disease into simple language.

After you have read this book, you should be provided with the information to relieve or even cure the most common symptom of acid reflux, heartburn, within eight to

twelve weeks, no matter how long you have suffered or how severe your condition.

Looking back on a medical practice of fifteen years, I am astonished by how much misinformation exists about therapies for stomach disorders. In part, this is because our knowledge of digestive diseases has increased so rapidly in the last two decades. In part, it is because of the slow-changing nature of medical practice. I too share this conservative approach to treatment and let the ancient Greek rule "First do no harm" govern my practice.

But not changing with the times can do harm as surely as staying with what was once thought to be safe and effective. And lack of patient knowledge can doom the efforts of even the most dedicated physician. Therapy is a team approach. Only by the continual exchange of information between patient and doctor can disease be controlled and eliminated.

I hope this book will encourage such dialogue and lead heartburn sufferers and health providers to examine carefully whether they are achieving the best available therapy. Any change in medication or lifestyle should be made in consultation with a physician. But all patients should carefully consider what the scientific evidence clearly shows us and the remarkable new pathways for relief and cure that have now opened.

—M. Michael Wolfe, M.D.,
Brigham and Women's Hospital
and Harvard Medical School

THE FIRE INSIDE

1

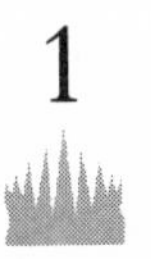

HEARTBURN

Fact and Myth

> The only way to keep your health is to eat what you don't want, drink what you don't like, and do what you'd druther not.
>
> —*Mark Twain*

Almost every day a heartburn patient who is fearful, confused, and in pain walks into my office. The pain and symptoms are sometimes unmistakable: a burning in the chest that spreads up the digestive tract into the sensitive lining of the gullet or esophagus. Other times the symptoms are confusing: wheezing, shortness of breath, chronic cough, and loss of voice.

All too often heartburn patients have spent years in a disappointing search for relief. The more typical patients, with the classic complaint of poor digestion and fiery lower throat, sometimes assume their condition is a normal part of eating and living. "The price we pay for bein' in the good old U.S.A." was how one of my patients put it. They usually come to see me because another doctor suspects an abnormality in their digestive tracts or because their pain has simply become unbearable.

Patients with less typical symptoms (or no symptoms of heartburn at all) sometimes come to my attention in unfortunate ways. Pat, a nurse in our hospital, suffered from severe asthma. This once-athletic woman had reached the point where she could barely walk, much less run her usual three miles a day. What saved her was a collapse on a Boston street corner and an ambulance race to the Brigham and Women's Hospital emergency room. While Pat was being examined, an internist discovered that she had an inflamed esophagus caused by acid reflux. Only then did she see me.

Odd as it may seem, many other sufferers with severe reflux disease also end up in the hospital emergency room. The most typical of these are seized with severe chest pain and believe they are having heart attacks. Sometimes they are put through a procedure to open the arteries before it is discovered that their disease originates in the stomachs, not in their blood vessels.

Once these patients have been referred to me, for whatever reason, my first job is to confirm that the problem stems from acid reflux. Sometimes we perform sophisticated tests; other times we simply start a course of therapy and see how patients respond. In nearly every case I need to calm the sufferer and explain that with modern therapy most people can expect to lead a virtually normal existence within a few months.

Pat, the Brigham and Women's Hospital nurse, recovered within six weeks of beginning antireflux therapy, after having been plagued with asthma for more than three years. She now breathes normally, no longer takes asthma medication, and has resumed a challenging routine of jogging. We'll discuss more about common lung, chest, and throat complications of acid disease in later chapters.

For now let's focus on another of my patients, Bill, a man who has symptoms of indigestion and burning of the esophagus with which most of us are familiar. As Bill graphically described his condition on his first visit, "Ever since I was a teenager, I've had this feeling like an erupting volcano was inside my chest." For years Bill had tried various remedies and was highly skeptical of ever finding relief.

When I first heard this, I simply nodded understandingly. I hear stories like this all the time from patients who think there is no hope and no help—even from medical specialists. So what could *I* do that's different? Let me admit that I'm not a miracle worker and don't have powers usually reserved for late-night television healers. What I do have is intense, personal experience treating stomach problems, the ability to recognize the source of many confusing symptoms, and a first-rate laboratory at the Brigham and Women's Hospital (one of the major medical centers affiliated with Harvard Medical School) that allows me to investigate the latest advances in gastroenterology. So I recognize that much of our information about treating heartburn and reflux disease is *very* new and that only recently have we understood what therapies are effective and how to use them.

Let me give you an example. In 1992 the *New England Journal of Medicine* published a study suggesting that surgery was superior to medicine in treating patients with severe acid reflux. This study is already out-of-date. New medicine, and better knowledge about the proper dosages of older medicines, now allow us to treat most severe reflux disease patients *without surgery*.

As recently as 1994 a major consumer advice magazine gave dangerous and incorrect information to its readers, one of whom happened to be my patient Bill.

This young man is exceptionally intelligent, curious, and funny. Indeed, he needed a sense of humor to stay on his job when, as he put it, "I felt like a blowtorch was scorching my gullet." Not only had Bill seen many physicians before me, but he had gone so far as to study medical books in our university library in an attempt to find a cure. (All he found were studies that were bewildering, contradictory, and controversial.) The physician who referred Bill to me was starting to believe that his patient knew more than he did.

It wasn't that Bill's symptoms were so unusual; it was how severe and persistent they were. He felt physical distress or burning after almost every meal. The fiery sensation surged up from his chest and into his esophagus. Bill was careful to avoid foods and liquids that irritated him, and he drank alcohol in moderation. Nonetheless, his life revolved around trips to the drugstore to buy antacids. "I go through rolls and rolls of them," Bill said. "Sometimes I feel like an addict. If a convenience store isn't in sight, I get the shakes."

After listening carefully to Bill's history of symptoms, I performed a routine test on him known as an endoscopy, which allows me to look down a patient's throat and into his esophagus with a long, flexible tube. The test showed nothing unusual. Bill's heartburn had not caused damage to the sensitive lining of any part of his throat.

It is extremely important to understand that *despite this lack of physical damage,* you may still have severe and painful heartburn. Don't let anyone rule out acid reflux just because physical abnormalities have not been detected. If you have symptoms—especially severe or bothersome ones—that is proof enough that the ailment is present. As I've said, heartburn is an extremely difficult disease to categorize. Only a fraction of sufferers seeks medical attention. Some of these people develop tiny ulcers or "erosions" in the esophagus; some develop the "masquerading" ailments we've spoken about. Sometimes symptoms are mild; other times they are severe. Odder still, physical damage, even severe physical damage to the throat and esophagus, can occur with none of the classic burning symptoms of heartburn. Another important point: Even if you have been diagnosed with the condition, do not assume that because you are taking heartburn medication, your disease is under control. If you continue to have symptoms, additional medical steps should be considered.

Like many others, Bill was already taking a prescription heartburn medication when he came to see me. This medicine, known as an H2 blocker, decreases the amount of acid produced in the stomach. Currently there are several such popular medications available, each of which works in a similar way. The first of these drugs to become available was called Tagamet, and others you may know include Zantac, Pepcid, or Axid. The term "H2 blocker" refers to the way these drugs "block" the production of stomach acid. They are the most commonly taken drugs in the world.

Many people with heartburn get relief shortly after taking these medications. However, many of these excellent drugs are prescribed at the *wrong* dosage or the wrong time of day for heartburn sufferers. That's because these medicines were originally used to treat stomach and duodenal ulcers. (The duodenum lies just below the stomach.) Often the dosage a heartburn patient needs is higher than the dosage a patient with a stomach or duodenal ulcer needs.

If you are currently taking one of these medications and not feeling as good as you think you should, do not decide to change your dosage by yourself. Discuss the problem with your doctor, as Bill did. I told him to take his pills three or four times a day, instead of twice, and to let me know if he started to feel better. He did get some relief, but not enough.

"I'm still in pain, and I'm still taking antacids," Bill told me a month after his treatment began. He was truly scared at this point because he thought surgery might be his only option.

I performed a more sophisticated test on Bill with a device known as a pH probe. The probe measures the degree of acidity of the stomach contents that are splashing against the esophagus, and it confirmed what Bill was telling me: Despite his increased medication, acidic food and stomach acid were still washing up his digestive tract.

However, instead of recommending surgery, instead of adding drugs to the one he was already taking, I prescribed a new capsule, a medicine called Prilosec. It is a drug that works by a different method and is more powerful than those existing before. In less than a week Bill's symptoms had disappeared. He was able to drink coffee; he had a few beers after work. He ate without pain. He slept through the night. In short, his life had changed. And he had to take the tablet only once a day.

Prilosec can also be used to diagnose your disease. If you live in an area where a pH probe is not available, your doctor may give you a dose of this drug as a test. Because Prilosec can markedly reduce the production of stomach acid, physicians sometimes prescribe it to see how well it eliminates symptoms. In medicine we call this empirical therapy, which is an elaborate way of saying, "If this drug eliminates your disease, that's the disease that probably affected you in the first place."

Actually, while I often perform the precise medical tests I used with Bill, most of the time I can make a near-perfect diagnosis by just listening to my patients like Mary, who said she had tried *everything*. And she had: antacids, prescription medications, massage therapy, chiropractic therapy, hydrotherapy, acupuncture—and a list of alternative healing methods stopping just short of voodoo and witchcraft. Because traditional medicine had offered Mary so little in the way of effective cures for her heartburn, she, like many others, turned to advice from everyone from her local hairdresser to her grandmother. I can almost tell how severe a patient's illness is by how many ineffective remedies he or she has tried. The more outlandish the treatments and the greater the number of relatives consulted, the worse the disease.

Mary had other sure signs of heartburn: She regarded spicy ethnic cuisine (which she loved), from Chinese to Mexican, with dread; she "snuck" pieces of chocolate, to her later regret; and she didn't dare sit, lie, or move in certain positions.

I can also gauge the severity of people's heartburn by asking about the number of bottles of antacids in their medicine chests. If the cabinets can be closed only by slamming them shut, I can make a very good start at a diagnosis.

Perhaps because of the odd and ineffective ways that heartburn has been treated, and the involuntary and embarrassing ways the disease can show itself, heartburn has been the source of a great deal of humor. The only book in the public library that refers specifically to heartburn is a novel by the comedy writer Nora Ephron, and it isn't about her medical condition, but about her marriage. Ms. Ephron's implied definition of heartburn, "as a painful, sometimes funny and confusing human condition," goes back at least to the fourteenth century, when Chaucer referred to single women as "brewing up herte-bren" for the town bachelors.

The public mistakes the symbolic meaning of the word "heartburn," which has long been used in the comic sense, with a very real, very painful, and sometimes very serious stomach acid-related illness. Patients receive the message that heartburn is a joke, or that it will quickly go away, or that it doesn't require treatment.

All untrue. In addition, the message about heartburn that patients have received has led them to be misinformed about its cause. Like characters in Nora Ephron's book, they come to my office with endless stories about what has given them heartburn: "bad husbands," "bad jobs," "bad traffic," "bad bosses"—or (in the case of one of my young female patients) "bad boys." I usually tell my patients the cause is more likely to be "bad luck."

Because while many of the nasty situations described by my patients probably didn't *help* their stomach problems, the situations themselves were not the basic cause of their illness.

Heartburn results from the fact that your body (through no fault of yours and for no particular reason) mixes acid and food in your stomach and launches it in the wrong direction. (Food and acid should go down, not up.) This irritating mixture is normally blocked from entering the esophagus by a protective barrier called a sphincter (see figure 1). Think of this protective barrier as a one-way swinging door. It is designed to allow food to go down but not to allow the digested, acidic remains of the food to come back up. When this

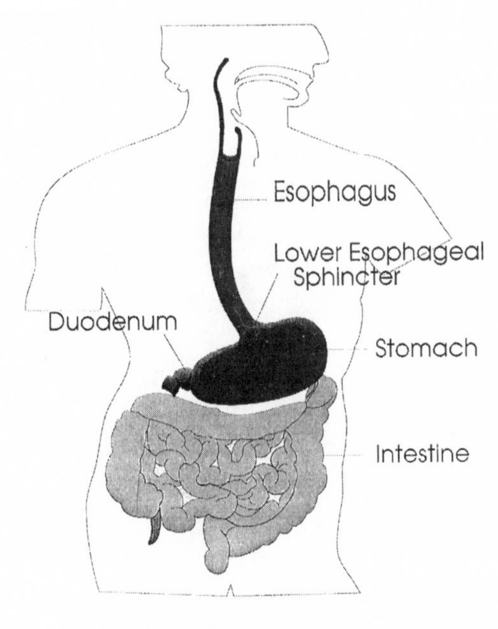

fig 1

barrier malfunctions, it fails to keep acid from flowing upward, or refluxing into the esophagus, causing a fiery sensation and sometimes tissue damage. You are more or less an innocent bystander in this process. Neither food, boys, girls, marriage, rush-hour traffic, or any other reality of life will alter this basic bodily problem.

Some people *are* more susceptible to the symptoms of the illness and should pay particular attention to this book. Eighty percent of pregnant women experience heartburn, and the incidence of the disease doubles over the age of fifty. Obesity, diet, other ailments, and medications are also likely factors. However, the disease can strike *anyone,* even newborns, and at one time or another *you* are likely to experience it.

If we know the cause of heartburn, why has its treatment been so difficult? Several reasons. As we've seen, the malady has such a broad range of symptoms and physical manifestations that it can be very hard to diagnose. In the people with typical symptoms the greatest difficulty is that most sufferers don't seek help from a physician. They either think that "indigestion is normal" or continue to deal with their pain with antacids. While antacids may work for mild and occasional heartburn, they have drawbacks. Antacids act for only a short period and thus must be taken constantly. This is impossible while sleeping during the night, and so patients find themselves waking in pain every few hours. (Another clue I use to diagnose my patients' heartburn is the dark circles under their eyes. The darker the circles from lack of sleep, the more severe the illness.)

My patient Bill rarely got a full night's rest. He thought it was normal to awaken every few hours to gulp antacids. But in fact, these medications were becoming a hazard. His stomach produced too much acid, and the barrier to his esophagus was too weak for an antacid to be of any benefit. Bill's condition became worse by his using antacids because while they partially helped his symptoms, they did not prevent acid from flowing *up* the food passageway.

As I stated, the most common prescription heartburn drugs, the H2 blockers—Tagamet, Zantac, Pepcid, and Axid—work well with many patients with *moderate* heartburn, but they take much more time to work than antacids. Thus some patients grow impatient with them. At the Brigham and Women's Hospital we are testing a new regimen that for the first time *unites* antacids with H2 blockers. For many heartburn sufferers, this may greatly help treatment. It allows patients to get rapid relief of symptoms (provided by antacids) and enduring relief (provided by H2 blockers). I will explain more about the basis for this therapy later in the book.

The important point to remember is that every person with heartburn needs to get the treatment that fits his or her condition. There is no *one correct* therapy, although there are many *incorrect* ones.

If you have a mild case of heartburn now and again, you may only need to eliminate or cut down on the foods we'll review in the next chapter or take an antacid. But if your symptoms are painful, if they are long-lasting, if they are starting to disrupt your life, getting medical attention is absolutely necessary.

I could describe hundreds of patients I've treated whose heartburn was so painful they could barely get through a day. A salesperson I knew could hardly speak and was starting to cancel important presentations; an executive assistant found it almost impossible to bend over to reach her files; a minister was becoming so hoarse he was unable to preach his weekly sermons. But you should be heartened to know that each of these patients has long since healed.

Unfortunately millions more have not. Because they did not get the right advice, continued with ineffective therapies, or did not take their conditions seriously, they went on to develop significant medical problems. Reflux disease is not a joke. In rare instances it can even be life-threatening. The constant flow of acid into areas near the esophagus, throat, and lungs can seriously damage these vital organs.

The fastest-growing cancer in the United States, cancer of the esophagus, may follow from acid reflux.

But it does not have to happen. If you learn nothing else from this book, it is that you do not have to live in pain and do not have to worry about developing complications. Not unless you ignore what is bothering you.

Now here's even more good news. Once you know the facts about heartburn and reflux disease, you're going to worry a lot less and feel a lot better. You won't have to avoid certain foods or keep popping pills that barely give you relief. You won't have to listen to your uncle Phil's jokes or try Grandmom's remedies.

You may even save yourself a great deal of money! The dollars you save on useless treatments may add up to the price of the banquet you thought you could never eat (much less afford).

The answers are all in this book. Enjoy!

2

SIMPLE HEARTBURN RELIEF

Lifestyle Modification

I have frequently known the heart-burn cured by chewing green tea.
—*William Buchan,* Domestic Medicine, *1789*

So much myth and lack of information surround the treatment of heartburn that most patients are unaware of the many simple ways the symptoms of the ailment can be relieved. And millions of sufferers don't know that understanding what aggravates heartburn may point them toward proper diagnosis and cure. A great deal of confusion seems to arise from the fact that certain normally healthful foods (such as fresh fruits) and activities (exercising) can either cause the typical burning heartburn symptom or bring on or increase the less well-known symptoms: hoarseness, chronic cough, or wheezing. Because of the chameleonlike nature of the Great Masquerader and the poor knowledge of its relationship to diet and activity, many patients put themselves on "strict" regimens, only to find themselves getting worse.

There's nothing new about going on the wrong diet or taking worthless medicine, as we shall see. In the case of heartburn, many links among foods, behavior changes, and acid-related disorders have only recently been proved or disproved by scientific investigation, and these findings are not well known by the public.

Heartburn is an age-old affliction, and remedies for it have been tried at least since the time of the ancient dwellers of Sumeria. The first written record of a heartburn treatment was made by the Roman scientist and historian Pliny the Elder, who recommended "coral powder." This compound contains calcium carbonate, an ingredient still used in many antacid formulations.

In the second century A.D. the Greek physician Galen first medically defined heartburn and devised a "remedy" that survived almost eighteen hundred years. Galen recognized that a common digestive complaint—"an uneasy burning sensation in the lower part of the chest"—might be connected with the region near the heart, and thus he termed the malady καρδιαλγία or kardialgia, "heart pain." The Latin term *cardialgia* ("heartburn") has survived to modern times, and physicians still sometimes find it a challenging task to differentiate between the pain of heartburn and the pain of heart attack. Galen's prescription for heartburn (and many other diseases) was called theriac, a potent brew of seventy compounds, the most noteworthy of which was the narcotic opium, another frequent ingredient in Greek medicine. Opium has the twofold advantage of dulling pain and inducing sleep. (Interestingly, until very recently, opium was often used to deal with the searing pain of stomach ulcer.)

Along with drugs, the ancient Greeks, among other peoples of the period, were aware that how individuals ate and lived affected their overall health. Greek physicians treated disease with diets of gruel, honey, vinegar, and water and generally recommended moderation in physical activity and sexual conduct. Modern physicians term this form of therapy lifestyle modification, and while specific medical recommendations may have changed, the reaction of patients to the various regimens imposed upon them has remained consistent.

Referring to doctors of his time, Pliny wrote: "There is alas no law against physician incompetency; no striking example is made. They learn by our bodily jeopardy and make experiments until the death of the patients, and the doctor is the only person not punished for murder." Obviously many remedies of the era were neither very popular nor very effective.

Over the centuries the search for more effective solutions to acid reflux continued. Through the years it seems that nearly every food, drug, or behavioral treatment was tried: herbs, powder of pearls, religious ceremonies, witchcraft, voodoo, cocaine, arsenic, and the application of leeches.

By the late 1800s the standard medical regimen for heartburn and indigestion had more or less come full circle from the Greco-Roman era: milk and antacids. The formula for their use was devised in the early part of the twentieth century by a doctor with the unlikely name of Bertram Sippy. The Sippy diet, which most patients believed referred to the bland liquid regimen, not the physician, consisted of hourly feedings of milk and antacids. The purpose of this diet was to counteract the destructive actions of stomach acids, which by that time were understood to be a cause of damage to the digestive tract.

The Sippy diet remained a mainstay of heartburn treatment until the early 1970s, when modern scientific investigation showed that the regimen was both unnecessary and a source of frequent side effects. On the other hand, when properly taken, antacids containing ingredients such as sodium bicarbonate, aluminum hydroxide, and various forms of magnesium do provide relief of heartburn symptoms in most patients with mild disease. They will not heal tissue damage or treat more serious presentations of heartburn. In chapter 3 we'll give the first complete review of how well antacids work, for whom they are most beneficial, the proper dosage, and side effects.

This information is not easily available because antacids were formulated and prescribed long before the Food and Drug Administration was mandated to require strict testing for drug safety *and* effectiveness. Today any medication used for heartburn must undergo extensive tests to see *if* it works, for how long, and in what patient groups. Specifically a new drug must be compared with an inactive "sugar pill," or placebo, to test if the new compound is any better than an inactive substance. This comparison eliminates what is known as the placebo effect, which occurs when patients get better (or worse) after ingesting a tablet containing nothing more than air, sugar, and water. If patients *believe* that a certain remedy relieves their symptoms, as many as 40 percent will improve, even if they are taking only sugar pills.

It's this fact that accounts for the continued use of and belief in the myriad dubious substances used to treat heartburn (including your uncle Phil's). If leeches are administered to patients, 40 percent of them will improve if they think leeches will help, and 40 percent will be relieved by chewing green tea or swallowing herbs. For now, let's return to nondrug approaches and see what steps can be taken to relieve mild heartburn without any medication at all.

As we've said, lifestyle modification—alteration of diet and behavior—was one of the first ways disease of any kind was treated. Surely the connection between diet and heartburn must have been noted early in human existence because by its nature most forms of "indigestion" cannot occur without some food substance to activate it. In the usual population food causes the stomach to produce most of its acid and ultimately bring harm to the body. Thus certain religious fasts and Spartan diets could very well have originated with some link to the serious illnesses associated with reflux disease. If an emperor suffered from asthma associated with severe acid indigestion, the asthma could possibly have been alleviated through a very restricted diet or a fast. Imagine the power and prestige a healer might have attained by restoring breath to the ruler.

It is remarkable, when we survey world medical literature, how similar medical advice has been regarding "overindulgence" and the encouragement of moderation. In the fourth century the Chinese physician Ko Hung wrote a treatise on prolonging life that might just as easily have been composed by any ancient doctor or modern practitioner: "Work without overexertion, eat in moderation especially before sleep, rise at cockcrow and end activity at sunset."

Good advice. But a difficult prescription in today's fast-paced, rapidly changing high-pressure world.

One of my patients, Ted, is a forty-seven-year-old Vietnam War veteran who works as a Boston police officer. When he is on a difficult case, his hours start at seven in the morning and don't end until after ten at night. Ted sometimes doesn't eat "breakfast" until noon, at which time he "gulps down" (as he puts it) a chocolate doughnut, pepperoni pizza, and coffee. He may not have dinner until midnight, when he eats a plate of takeout fried chicken, potato salad, and coleslaw with two beers while watching the Letterman show. On his last visit to my office Ted described his heartburn as a "catastrophe" and asked me, in all seriousness, what could *possibly* be causing his problem.

I guess I could have said, "Beats the hell out of me," and ordered a half dozen expensive tests, but as you've guessed, it really wasn't necessary. So in order to understand Ted and his fellow sufferers, let's start with the process of eating.

It begins with the chewing of food or, with increasing numbers of rushed individuals, with the gulping or inhaling of it. In any case, food placed in the mouth mixes with saliva and soon starts down the food passageway or digestive tract. It is, naturally, helpful to *swallow* first (if you have time) to move the food and saliva mixture downward.

Everything you've done thus far, including your choice of pizza topping, has been voluntary, but as food moves down to the esophagus, the process of digestion becomes involuntary. Heartburn occurs because the lining of the esophagus is very sensitive (much more so than the lining of the stomach) and can be irritated both by the acid normally found in some foods and by the acid splashing up from the stomach. In addition, anything that *delays* the journey of this washed-up food and acid out of the esophagus will cause further damage and increase the burning symptoms of heartburn.

At the lower end of the esophagus, as previously shown, there is a valve or sphincter, like a one-way swinging door, that allows food to continue moving down the digestive tract but prevents it from coming back up. The body accomplishes this with a complex system of chemical signals that can be affected by such factors as food, medication, and physical exertion. The chemical signals both cause the "door" or valve to open and cause it to close and stay shut. When this valve beneath the esophagus allows food to pass upward too easily, we refer to it as "relaxed."

Some people say they have "ironclad stomachs" and never experience heartburn. These fortunate souls have strongly resistant linings of their food passageways and are very efficient at digesting food. They can eat and drink anything—even while racing to catch a train—and still feel fine. At the other extreme are people who get heartburn simply by thinking of food. In these people the linings of the digestive tract are very sensitive and the junction between the stomach and esophagus is virtually *always* relaxed.

While my patient Ted is someone whose diet and lifestyle are a "model" for inducing heartburn, many others like him will never experience the malady. On the other hand, many of my patients live calm and normal lives, eat regular healthy meals, and experience heartburn every bit as painful and debilitating as Ted's. Heartburn is an individual matter, and what affects one person may not affect another. And so many foods and medications have been associated with heartburn that it may be very difficult and sometimes impossible to avoid them all.

In the first category of heartburn irritants are foods and drugs that cause the one-way door or valve at the base of the esophagus to "relax" and open at the wrong times. The most common foods that create this problem are those high in fat or containing caffeine: chocolate and soft drinks (like Dr Pepper or Coke). Coffee, whether it is caffeinated or decaffeinated, is one of the most commonly consumed substances in this category. Countless patients assure me that they drink only "decaf." However, a 1975 study in the *New England Journal of Medicine* conclusively proved that decaffeinated coffee is almost as potent as regular coffee in both stimulating stomach acid production and causing the esophageal valve to relax.

Coffee lovers will not enjoy hearing that the coffee bars that are springing up like weeds around the country are wonderful for conversation and meeting new friends but not at all helpful for heartburn. The various combination coffee drinks, containing steamed milk and chocolate (among other ingredients), can truly be irritating.

"But I *love* these drinks!" I hear you saying.

Yes, I know. But each item in them is known to aggravate heartburn and may leave you feeling miserable soon after the first pleasant sips. In fact, if you would like to make your coffee drink even *more* incendiary, add some mint to the chocolate. In another study to determine the foods associated with heartburn, it was shown that peppermint oil (and all the foods that contain it) also relaxes the valve between the esophagus and stomach. So after-dinner mints, especially those covered with chocolate, are among the *worst* after-dinner foods. Ironically, they are often left on the pillows of hotel rooms to make sure guests get a good night's sleep.

Breath fresheners that contain mint will not improve

your social life. Popping them before a date can give heartburn sufferers indigestion all evening and cause reflux that will induce a bad odor in the mouth!

Some people manage to make their heartburn *worse* when they change certain foods in their diet. That was the case with one of my patients whose mild and occasional heartburn was growing more severe. He was otherwise in excellent health and extremely careful about his diet, but something was causing his distress. I finally learned that after he had given up coffee of any kind, he had started substituting herbal teas, one of which was a potent brew of assorted mint leaves. It never occurred to the patient that this "health drink" could worsen his heartburn symptoms.

Other drinks that have this effect are those containing alcohol: from wine, beer, and bourbon to champagne and cognac. It's not the quality of the liquor but the chemical components that count. Experiments on healthy subjects have shown that alcohol in sufficient quantity stimulates production of acid and relaxes the valve between the stomach and esophagus. Lastly, cigarette smoking, and nicotine in particular, may irritate the lining of the throat and disrupt normal digestion.

Dairy products promote heartburn by increasing the stimulation of acid in the stomach and by increasing the length of time the washed-up acid stays in contact with the esophagus. Therefore, many people with heartburn should avoid milk, cheeses, ice cream, and yogurt—especially those that are high in fat.

In the final category of "heartburn-provoking foods" are items with high acid contents. These foods directly irritate the lining of the digestive tract and cause additional acid to accumulate in the stomach. Good examples of such foods are citrus fruits (lemons, oranges, grapefruits), tomatoes, onions, and spices.

If you keep in mind all the foods I've referred to, you can see why certain popular nourishments are particularly lethal: pizza with sausage (spices, fat, cheese, and tomatoes); lasagna; salads with "ranch" dressing and Caesar salads (grated cheese, egg yolk, lemon juice, and fried bread); fried chicken and Big Mac lunches. In fact, if you can eat a hamburger with bacon, cheese, pickles, onions, mayonnaise, and fries and still *not* get heartburn, you can probably safely eat anything.

This food list is neither complete nor definitive and is intended only as a general guide. It seems that each of my heartburn patients has a particular food that causes problems. What irritates one person with heartburn may not irritate another, and sensitivities may also vary according to the quantity of substances consumed. You may be fine with one cup of coffee, but not with two. Individual tolerance is important here.

Some patients seem to improve overnight simply by cutting down on or eliminating coffee, mints, and caffeinated soft drinks. Other patients have greatly improved by lowering the fat in their diets and avoiding fried foods. Low-acid tomatoes are worth considering, and make your sauce without onions and very little oil. Use low-fat accompaniments to your pasta (mushrooms instead of meat sauce), and be careful not to pile butter, cheese, sour cream, and bacon bits on top of a baked potato. Green salads are healthy, but don't saturate them with high-fat dressings. You'll feel better and lose weight!

A word of caution: *Do not undertake any dietary therapy without first consulting a physician.* If you experience continuing pain after eating, you should have the problem evaluated. *Patients with severe heartburn will rarely be helped simply by diet changes.*

Another group of substances associated with heartburn are various prescription and nonprescription medications. Making changes in these cases can be a considerable challenge. One of the most difficult problems occurs among asthmatics. As I've explained, not only can reflux disease bring on an attack of asthma, but the medications used to treat asthma, such as theophylline (Theo-Dur), can worsen acid disease. As a result, patients are caught in a cycle in which both asthma and reflux escalate as more asthma medication is prescribed. Theophylline not only relaxes the digestive valve but increases acid production by the stomach. This problem may be helped by using a lower dosage of the asthma drug or an alternate form of therapy, such as an inhaled steroid. Another class of asthma drugs, beta 2-adrenergic drugs (Ventolin or Proventil), has been shown to increase heartburn somewhat when taken orally but rarely when taken as an inhalant.

Patients with high blood pressure and heart disease must be particularly careful if they also have heartburn. Remember that doctors of antiquity associated heartburn with heart disease, and in some ways the two ailments mimic each other. Ironically, medication that relieves the pain of heart illness may worsen heartburn. Specifically, calcium channel blockers, such as Cardizem and Procardia, can cause adverse effects on digestion. *However, if you have reason to believe you are in any danger of heart disease, always put that consideration first*. Indigestion can indeed be a symptom of a heart attack.

Other drugs can aggravate acid disease. These include aspirin and other nonsteroidal anti-inflammatory drugs, such as Advil or Nuprin, birth control pills, and other medications with estrogen, such as Premarin, commonly given to postmenopausal women.

If you have heartburn and are taking one of these medications, consult your doctor and see if an alternative can be worked out. If none can be found, you will most likely need to take specific medicines to prevent acid disease from damaging your body. *Do not change your medical regimen in any way without first talking to your doctor.*

It may seem at this point that only "bad" things cause heartburn. (I define a "bad thing" as something everyone's mother tells him or her not to eat or do.) Unfortunately other forms of lifestyle changes that are beneficial under normal circumstances may also lead to increased episodes and severity of heartburn. For example, studies show that physical exertion increases the likelihood of upward acid flow. These reports prove that jogging induces heartburn symptoms in otherwise healthy individuals, and in one study of fifty-two patients, twenty-three, or almost one half, felt heartburn distress while on a treadmill.

In real life this means that in heartburn-prone people, a "healthy" jog or even a vigorous walk after dinner can bring on a feeling of having a heart attack. This happened to my aunt. She is an energetic woman in her late seventies who always takes an evening walk. One night after returning home, she felt an uneasy sensation in her chest. As the pain worsened, she became convinced she was having a heart attack. Fortunately she wasn't; she was undergoing a severe episode of heartburn that was successfully treated with medicine.

In my aunt's case the situation was made worse by a very simple action. After her exercise she lay down on her bed to rest. In people with normal digestion there would be no reaction. But among people with reflux disease, lying down helps bring on *heartburn* symptoms. About half the people with chronic heartburn pump more acid into the esophagus when prone. Many of these people could get relief just by sitting up and letting the force of gravity help move food *down* the digestive tract. When heartburn sufferers lie flat, more food remains in the stomach, thus producing more acid that rises into the esophagus. Lying down also causes stomach acid to remain in contact longer with sensitive digestive tract linings.

This problem becomes worse at night, just when you're climbing into bed to read or watch television. During these hours your body decreases its flow of saliva; without saliva, the esophagus is irritated even more.

A simple helpful trick is to use some lozenges, sucking candy, or gum. These items stimulate saliva, which contains a natural antacid that can counteract the effect of acid in your esophagus. Only a small increase in salivary fluid can sometimes do the job.

Another solution is not to lie down for two or three hours after eating a meal. This is especially true after the evening meal, which in the United States tends to be heavier than breakfast or lunch and occurs closer to bedtime. If you're going to take a siesta after a meal, it's better to do it in a reclining chair or, as people in many countries do, in a semisitting position.

Another helpful technique is to elevate the head of the bed with three- to six-inch blocks so that you sleep on a slight incline. Just propping your head up on pillows will not do any good; it will only make your heartburn more painful. Your *entire* upper digestive tract needs to be raised.

While scientific experiments have documented the

beneficial medical effects of inclining the bed, there may be unpredictable social consequences. It is very unsettling to have your spouse slide to the foot of the bed, for example. One of my colleagues recommended blocks to a patient and asked at the next visit how he was doing. "Oh, I'm doing fine," the patient said. "But my wife fell on the floor and sprained her ankle."

To avoid putting your relationships in jeopardy, you can purchase a firm foam wedge that elevates you from the waist and is just as effective as elevating the entire bed. One such foam wedge is called the Bedge. (See the appendix for further information. Other devices similar to the Bedge are now available in many shops.)

During the day you can easily make changes in the way you position your body. Bend at the knees rather than at the waist when you pick up an object. Bending at the waist increases pressure in your stomach and forces up acid.

Actually any pressure against the digestive tract provokes heartburn. I have seen patients improve dramatically just by loosening their clothes. One perplexing case I recently encountered was with a young woman, Ellen, who had just started dating. I could find absolutely nothing wrong with her, but after discussions I learned that Ellen's heartburn occurred only when she saw her new boyfriend. He "adored her" in tight jeans, and my patient complied by wearing garments so restrictive I was amazed she could walk in them. The story has a happy ending all around. Ellen's boyfriend apparently liked her just as much in loose-fitting clothes, and not only did Ellen's romance bloom, but her heartburn disappeared.

The moral: If possible, both men and women should avoid constricting garments, especially binding undergarments. If you must wear restricting clothes to work (a uniform, business suit, etc.), change when you get home into a robe or stretch clothes.

Finally it is helpful to lose weight. While we do not exactly understand how, obesity is associated with heartburn, and losing weight often goes along with relief of heartburn symptoms. Studies in this regard are not very encouraging because few people manage lasting weight loss. But it may help you to stay on your diet to know that not only will you look better, but you will probably notice a marked relief in your heartburn symptoms. The antiheartburn diet is very similar to the low-cholesterol diet and in line with the nutritional guidelines of the federal government.

Knowing what causes heartburn should help you find ways of easing it. For example, now that you know the consequences of food staying longer in the system, you can understand why eating large meals causes irritation. Big meals take longer to digest and force the stomach to produce more acid. You can also understand why "eating on the run" is harmful, as body movement can precipitate acid reflux. The body requires a certain amount of time to perform the crucial task of converting food into useful substances. As you speed up, your body's digestive system slows down.

Having given you this advice, I need to explain that while doctors who work at Harvard are often thought of as living in an ivory tower, it is a tower with an excellent view of Boston. People and cars rush by or crawl to a frustrating halt in rush-hour traffic. Doctors within the "tower" must spring up from the lunchroom, food in hand, to cope with emergency phone pages.

Under these circumstances, when many of us are overwhelmed by job and family pressures, why even recommend lifestyle modifications? Many reasons. They have no cost and no side effects, and best of all, the changes will benefit your general health. For some people, just making small conduct changes or being aware of symptom-inducing foods, drugs, and behaviors can help them devise regimens that will relieve their pain. Just as important, if you have any of the "silent" heartburn problems that signal more severe disease, knowing the foods that cause aggravation can guide you toward a diagnosis and cure. For example, does your hoarseness get worse with coffee or alcohol? Do mints or fatty foods cause more wheezing?

If your lifestyle continues to present you with pain that is difficult or impossible to alter, other measures are available, beginning with antacids and more potent prescription and nonprescription drugs. You will have to find your own balance between the way you wish to live and the medications that will allow you to live it.

3

ACID AND ANTACID

Magnesia has long been a celebrated remedy for stomach complaints.

—Medical Journal II, *1799*

What is life without chicken paprikash?

—*Uncle Harry*

Although for centuries the wide array of disorders and symptoms associated with reflux disease was well known, the fact that the workings and contents of the digestive tract could not be seen gave rise to every imaginable belief about the causes and cures of acid reflux. Most peculiarly no one could see any actual signs of damage to the body, so how serious could the disease be? The symptoms were certainly unbearable, but what was causing them? The planets? Bad vapors? Certain foods? Or as one nineteenth-century physician suggested, "French novels"?

Only recently have we have made two simple yet profound discoveries. Serious and even life-threatening reflux disease can take place without obvious physical damage to the body. As you may recall, this was the case with my patient Bill. He and other people with acid reflux have symptoms of heartburn, chest pain, and asthma, but no injury to the esophagus or adjacent organs. In other words, the pain occurs without any observable harm to the body.

Secondly, for the most part the actual physical damage done by reflux disease can be detected only by sophisticated diagnostic equipment. A physician cannot detect acid reflux using normal diagnostic tools found in the usual clinic or office during a physical examination.

We have also learned that the root cause of reflux disease is something that seems obvious and ordinary: stomach acid. But don't be deceived. We are only now beginning to understand the complex process by which stomach acid is manufactured and utilized and what causes it to do so much harm when it escapes from the organ in which it was intended to stay.

No matter what symptoms of reflux disease you are experiencing—from mild heartburn to intense chest pain—your most basic problem is an extremely potent corrosive compound. Even voice loss and asthma may well be linked to the constant wearing away or "corrosive" effect of stomach acid moving into parts of your body where it can easily do damage. Not only can this eroding action cause continual and painful symptoms, but the inflammation associated with stomach acid irritation may eventually lead to cancer. In fact, cancers of various parts of the digestive tract (like the esophagus) are the fastest-growing malignancies in the United States.

If the basis of our suffering is a body substance as well known and easily identifiable as stomach acid, you would think that the medical solution would be simple: a substance that tames or neutralizes the harmful effects of stomach acid.

In fact, such substances are now readily available to all of us. They take up entire aisles in our drugstores and line the shelves of our supermarkets. Their brand names—Mylanta, Maalox, Tums, Rolaids—are as familiar to us as Coke and Pepsi, and they are *regularly* consumed by at least one third of the adult population of the United States.

So why does so much suffering continue? Why does acid-related disease still remain so destructive? If the problem is stomach acid, why can't antacids, which are convenient, plentiful, and relatively safe and inexpensive compounds, solve all our problems?

There are many answers. First, most patients do not understand the proper use and limitations of these drugs. They are often taken at incorrect doses, at the wrong time of day, and for too long a period. In some cases they cause harmful side effects or conceal various medical problems of which patients may be completely unaware. The directions on most antacid bottles can be misleading because their recommendations are too broad. As we've seen, acid-related diseases cover an enormously wide spectrum of illness, from mild to life-threatening. If this book did nothing else, I would be very pleased if it informed millions of consumers about the how, when, and why of antacid use.

Another reason why antacids have their limitations is that heartburn and many of the related diseases are likely to be chronic problems. They bother us nearly all the time—or at least frequently enough to interfere with many of our ordinary daily activities. But antacids are recommended only for people who have *occasional* and *mild* illness. That is one of the proper precautions described on the medication labels. Antacids should not be used every day and become part of your daily routine like brushing your teeth.

Nonetheless, at least five to ten million Americans use antacids frequently—and for months or years at a time. What can happen? Recently I saw a forty-two-year-old man named Gary who had developed mild heartburn symptoms in his early thirties. Nothing serious, Gary had thought at the time, and he began to use antacids. As his heartburn symptoms became worse, he gradually increased the dose of his medication. This gave him temporary relief, but he was always tired and noticed an increasing shortness of breath and wheezing. Finally Gary developed full-blown asthma and an intense pressure in his chest that made him seek medical attention. By this time he was swallowing a pack of antacid tablets every day and avoiding almost all exercise. After I examined him, I found that Gary had a severe inflammation of his esophagus.

How unusual is Gary's case? We don't know for sure, but it may be more common than suspected. A recent report has confirmed that among heavy users of antacids, more than 30 percent had damage to the lining of their gullets. A small but significant number had dangerous (precancerous) ulcers in their esophagi. While researchers have not studied a large enough number of patients to reach a definitive conclusion, we suspect—because of the sheer number of people who suffer from heartburn and the enormous number of antacid users—that *millions* of people are at medical risk. I'll emphasize this over and over: Antacids are excellent drugs for relieving *occasional* symptoms of mild heartburn. They act rapidly and often effectively, and we should not toss out our antacid bottles or start to panic because we take Tums after figuring out our income taxes. But all of us should keep Gary's story in mind: Antacids rarely, if ever, heal tissues that have been inflamed or injured by stomach acid.

This probably seems surprising. An "antacid," as the name implies, is supposed to "counteract acid." It is supposed to make a destructive chemical harmless, and the fact that in many people it does accounts for the extraordinary popularity of these compounds. But in a significant number of sufferers, antacids are not sufficient because stomach acid is far stronger, more corrosive and dangerous than most people realize.

I learned about this misconception when I was teaching a group of first-year medical students. (Believe me, they didn't know much more about the composition of the stomach than does the average American.) The students were astonished by a simple demonstration of just how potent stomach acid is. I showed them a piece of thick paper, then dipped it into a jar containing stomach acid. The paper actually burned and decomposed in the fluid. If you were to drip stomach acid on a piece of human skin, the same corrosive disintegration would take place.

Stomach or gastric juice contains hydrochloric acid, a powerful acid that is stored in special containers in my lab. It can be made harmless by pouring in the chemicals found in antacids. These "neutralizing" chemicals, in an almost instant reaction with the acid, create a harmless liquid that will not irritate a baby's bottom. But the more acid in the container, the more neutralizer you need. Without enough neutralizer the acid compound will still have the power to do damage.

What does this basic chemistry lesson have to do with your misery? Everything.

Within your stomach is a corrosive chemical that can easily destroy human tissue. What saves you is that your stomach is a remarkable organ that is designed to handle this powerful acid. As long as you have a healthy stomach and acid stays where it is supposed to, your body has no difficulty and you feel no pain. But when the acid surges upward from its natural resting place and is not blocked by the sphincter, you are left open to the destructive, burning reactions caused by a powerful chemical: Your chest burns; you wheeze; you become hoarse and lose your voice; you may develop lung inflammation and asthma or actually have a hole burned in your esophagus.

Or, as my patients put it, "A fire is inside."

No wonder that trying to tame stomach juice has been an age-old quest, and no wonder, because of the potency of the acid within, that the quest has been only partially successful.

Historians do not know exactly when the first antacids were discovered, but as previously mentioned, they were well known thousands of years ago. No one understood how they worked; the composition of stomach "juices" and how they functioned in the body were not understood until the nineteenth century. But as often happens in medicine, simple observation made it apparent that certain substances were easing the pain of heartburn and its associated ailments.

These "antacid" substances were presumed to work with a little help from mystical sources. For example, let's look back at the remedy used by Chinese doctors of the seventh century. Their cure for heartburn consisted of thick yellow paper containing magic characters inscribed with colored chemicals. These chemicals (which were embedded on the yellow paper) were very similar to our current antacids. The red substances contained mercuric oxide, the brown contained ferrous oxide, and the white contained calcium and magnesium carbonate.

After putting a spell on the cure, the physician burned the paper, and the patient was asked to consume the ashes along with a few particles of the chemical mixed with hot water. In short, the seventh-century Chinese were prescribing an ages-old precursor of milk of magnesia mixed with food coloring and help from supernatural sources.

The science of chemistry was a long way off, but doctors essentially recognized a basic principle: Certain substances are capable of rendering destructive elements in the body relatively harmless. We call these substances alkali or bases. When an alkali is mixed with an acid—whether it is mild acid like lemon juice or a powerful acid like that found in your stomach—the acid loses its destructive power. Alkaline substances include forms of magnesium, calcium, aluminum, and sodium. Toss these substances into a flask of hydrochloric acid, and the combined resulting liquid will no longer burn skin. Put them in your body, with or without magic numbers, and an almost immediate chemical reaction takes place that can make stomach acid harmless (neutral) and relieves your symptoms.

The problem doctors faced until very recently was that it often took more alkali than a patient could possibly consume to neutralize stomach acid completely. Thus horoscopes, numerology, and "magical ingredients" were called upon to heal the patient. (Indeed, even today many of my patients and not a few colleagues call for the help of a "higher authority" when confronting severe heartburn.)

This divine plea occurred through history whether the physician was Chinese, Arab, or European. In the sixteenth century, as modern Western medicine was evolving, the father of pharmacology, a doctor known as Paracelsus, developed a marvelous brew for relieving heartburn. He called this potion an amalgam because its miracle ingredient was magnesium (a related word). Paracelsus firmly believed in the influence of the stars and planets on physical health and was deeply involved in the world of the occult. The potion did seem to work often enough, so we can conclude that just as in China, patients were getting relief from their rudimentary Maalox.

During and after the Renaissance physicians began to look inside the body for answers to medical problems, rather than heavenward to astrology and numerology. The world of alchemy was evolving into the science of chemistry, and understanding was growing about the composition of the human body, including the nature of the juices inside the stomach. No one knew what they were exactly, but it was rapidly becoming evident that they could be lethal. In the sixteenth century, as the legal restrictions against performing autopsies lifted, physicians discovered that the stomach could be "eaten away," bleed, and cause death. A seventeenth-century scientist noted that digestion began in the stomach by "acid fermentation," and there was much debate about how this organ worked. "Was it a mill, a fermenting wine vat, or a stewpan?" one physician wondered. The problem was that no one could actually *look inside* the body to learn the answer. The best anyone could do was guess.

That is, until the early nineteenth century, at which time there occurred one of the most bizarre incidents in medical history. In 1822 an American frontier army surgeon of no particular distinction (and no formal medical training) was called to treat a French Canadian who was dying of a shotgun blast to the stomach. Dr.

William Beaumont looked inside his patient and clearly saw the badly damaged chest, lungs, and abdomen. Beaumont cleaned the wound, tried to make his patient as comfortable as possible, and "waited for the inevitable." But much to everyone's astonishment the patient lived, although the gaping hole in his body remained, and for ten years Beaumont used his patient as a living observational laboratory, eventually publishing a work entitled *Experiments and Observations on the Gastric Juice and the Physiology of Digestion.*

For the first time scientists knew through direct observation the composition of the stomach and how it worked. Beaumont described how food was digested by a complex series of chemical reactions, confirmed that stomach or gastric juices contained the powerful hydrochloric acid, and discovered that the amount of acid the body produced was related to the mental state of the patient. He also confirmed that most stomach acid isn't actually produced until food enters the digestive tract.

Now armed with a more concrete understanding of the stomach and its acids, nineteenth-century physicians experimented with new regimens (rest cures and starvation diets) and looked at ways of purifying and combining various foods and alkalies (antacids) to counteract further the destructive effect of acid. One fact was rapidly becoming evident, and in some ways it is the most important piece of information you need to know about your illness: If stomach acid is eliminated or greatly reduced in your body, its power to do damage decreases and digestive disease may be relieved.

But how do you remove a key part of the body's chemistry? How do you control the elemental process that turns our food to useful nutrients and still keep the patient functioning?

No one knew.

Many trends in eighteenth- and nineteenth-century society accompanied the development of science and medicine. The Industrial Revolution made it possible to grow and harvest more crops, distribute them to more people, and in greater quantities than had ever before been possible. Railroads were able to rush food grown and processed in one region of the country to every other; people moved from farms to overcrowded, unhygienic cities; the pace of life itself increased, and speed became an object of worship.

Stomach acid worked overtime.

"Dyspepsia is a disease of civilization," noted two nineteenth-century doctors. "All civilizations suffer from it, but none so much as the people of the United States." Much was made of this "modern epidemic." Physicians surmised that much of the cause was "gluttony," but nineteenth-century attitudes toward eating (and a good deal else) were highly ambivalent.

For at about the time that medical science experimented with rest and alkali cures for acid-related diseases, a notorious entrepreneur and gourmand called Diamond Jim Brady made headlines because of the amount of food he consumed. Often accompanied by the famous two-hundred-pound actress and singer Lillian Russell, Brady began a day with hominy, eggs, corn bread, muffins, flapjacks, chops, fried potatoes, a beefsteak, and a full gallon of orange juice. (You will recall from the previous chapter that this is not the lifestyle we recommend to counteract heartburn.)

As his nickname implied, Diamond Jim was a man fond of wealth and extravagance, but he was not alone. While he was reveling in New York, the corpulent William Howard Taft was elected president. At five feet eleven and 325 pounds, Taft holds the distinction of having been the nation's heaviest president. (When he moved into the White House in 1909, plumbers had to build a special bathtub to accommodate his girth.)

Perhaps not coincidentally, at the same time a physician in Chicago, Dr. Bertram Sippy, was developing a remedy for digestive problems that was to be the mainstay of treatment for many acid-related diseases in the twentieth century. Sippy subtitled his research paper "Medical Cure by an Efficient Removal of Gastric Juice Corrosion." In other words, he was trying to do what physicians had attempted for thousands of years: completely neutralize the acid in the stomach.

When we look at Sippy's regimen today, we can readily understand why past physicians resorted to chants, spells, and numerology to increase their odds of healing. Sippy's patients had to remain in hospital beds for four weeks. They were initially fed three ounces of milk and cream every hour from 7:00 A.M. to 7:00 P.M., then after a few days were allowed soft eggs and well-cooked cereals. Antacids were given to the patients between each feeding. Sippy maintained that this regimen controlled stomach acid and healed his patients, and the medical world accepted the finding.

What was the antacid that Sippy used? You may have guessed already. Magnesium. The same mineral to which the sixteenth-century Paracelsus had ascribed occult powers.

Sippy's Chicago team went on to experiment with other alkalies or antacids, and it wasn't long before the one-billion-dollar antacid market was off and running. By that time Diamond Jim was long in his grave and Taft had left politics.

Although Sippy and his team prescribed antacids for the control of stomach ulcers, most people take these drugs for reflux disease and its prime symptom, heartburn. This fact remains the source of a great deal of confusion among both patients and physicians. Stomach ulcer is not the same as reflux disease, although it is in the same family of acid-related diseases. The two entities are largely confused because the therapy for both is *deceptively* similar, their symptoms can be somewhat alike, and both illnesses are exacerbated by the corrosive effects of stomach acid.

It is important to understand that a stomach ulcer, as the name implies, affects the stomach and in most cases is caused by a combination of acid *remaining in the stomach* and a recently discovered and treatable infection with a bacterium known as *Helicobacter pylori*. Reflux disease is caused by acid *leaving* the stomach and affecting other parts of the body. It has no relationship to H. pylori and will not respond to antibiotics. Both illnesses *are* "acid-related," and without the corrosive effects of this chemical, neither can occur.

But despite popular perception, the two diseases are equally serious. It is just as harmful to have acid eating away your esophagus, lungs, throat, or voice box as it is your stomach. And reflux disease may have far greater complications when you consider that it may lead to cancer.

Part of the confusion about acid reflux or heartburn stems from the vague terms we use to describe our stomach problems: indigestion, stomach upset, queasiness—or, as doctors are prone to say, nonulcer dyspepsia. According to the *Handbook of Nonprescription Drugs*, this condition "refers to intermittent upper abdominal discomfort, the cause of which is not clearly defined." In other words, an occasional stomachache.

Because much of our abdominal distress, of whatever disease category, is caused by some kind of acid irritation, antacids and similar medications tend to be taken for just about every kind of stomach upset.

Remember, though, that true gastroesophageal reflux disease and its prime symptom, heartburn, involve a specific bodily malfunction that allows stomach juices to shoot upward. It is possible to have many vague forms of stomach upset and not to have this specific disease.

This fact relates to antacids because you cannot know which medicine to take and how much of it will be effective unless you know what your illness is. You cannot treat an ulcer the same way you treat reflux disease. You cannot treat mild heartburn the same way you treat severe chest pain. That's why we continually counsel you to get a physical examination if stomach distress, wheezing, shortness of breath, or chest pain persists or starts interfering with daily living.

Before we discuss how to use antacids, let's take a closer look at what's in all those colorful bottles and packets. As we've seen, various forms of the basic ingredients of modern antacids have been used for centuries.

But today's commercial products are actually very different from the brews, chalks, and powders of previous eras. All antacids contain at least one of four active ingredients: sodium bicarbonate, calcium, magnesium, and aluminum. When these ingredients were first given to patients, their quality, quantity, and purity were not assured. Furthermore, no one knew how to mix them together to minimize their side effects. Today our medications go through rigorous safety procedures so that we no longer have to worry about contamination or variation in dosage strength. We know exactly how much of each ingredient is in each liquid or tablet.

Every dose of a modern commercial antacid contains exactly the same amount of chemicals as every other.

This is extremely important because it allows you and your doctor to experiment to find the most effective amount of medicine for your condition. Remember the example of the acid in the glass container. We have to know how much is in it before we can figure out how much antacid it will take to render it harmless. Each person is unique. A tablespoon of antacid may work for one person but be far too little for another. Therefore, knowing exactly how much and what combinations of active ingredient are in each product is critical.

Let's now look at the most popular antacid preparations:

Sodium Bicarbonate or Baking Soda

The word "soda," which for most people now means a soft drink like Pepsi or 7-Up, originally referred to a sodium salt like soda ash. Soda water was the name given to a stomach medication that combined this soda (sodium salt) with carbonic acid ("carbonated water"). Soda fountains became popular in drugstores, where pharmacists could create fizzing soda water medicines and sometimes mix in other flavoring ingredients (cherry, lemon-lime, orange) to make the concoctions more tasty. (One of the most popular soda waters was created in part from syrup from the cola nut and eventually became the widely known "medicine" Coca-Cola.)

The most popular brands of medications that contain sodium bicarbonate are Alka-Seltzer and Bromo-Seltzer. These medications get their name from a German town called Niederselters that became famous for a natural sparkling water rich in sodium chloride. Conveniently the water also contains traces of magnesium and calcium. Pharmacists used their soda fountains to create copies of this German water, which became known as seltzer, and sold it as an aid to digestion.

Sodium-containing compounds have the advantage of being inexpensive, rapid, and effective. But sodium may be dangerous for people with high blood pressure or on a (sodium-) salt-restricted diet. A pinch of baking soda mixed with water is very safe and can rapidly extinguish an attack of heartburn, but sodium compounds should *not* be used on a regular basis or in high doses.

People with stomach problems should be particularly careful about Alka-Seltzer. This product unfortunately combines sodium bicarbonate with aspirin. Aspirin is a known stomach irritant (in fact, aspirin is itself an acid) and can also damage the small intestine. In some people aspirin can wear down the stomach lining that normally protects us from acid and leave the stomach and small intestine susceptible to ulcers. Therefore, if you are prone to stomach problems, I do not recommend this product.

Calcium-Based Antacids (Tums, Alka-2, Titralac)

Calcium carbonate is fast-acting and potent. The compound is a white powder made from chalk, bones, and shells and was widely used by German physicians in the middle 1800s and later as part of Dr. Sippy's regimen. Like sodium-based antacids, these compounds are good in low doses for short-term relief but should not be used in higher doses or long term.

Too much calcium (like sodium bicarbonate) can damage the kidneys and lead to calcium deposits in the eyes and skin. Ironically, it was the Sippy diet that brought attention to this side effect and was one of the reasons it fell out of favor. Another problem with calcium-based compounds is that while they initially work and neutralize stomach acid, calcium itself can stimulate stomach acid.

So what do we recommend? Calcium is an essential mineral for healthy bones and teeth and to prevent osteoporosis in postmenopausal women. Taking just one calcium-containing antacid tablet a day will help prevent this serious bone disease if taken prior to the onset of menopause. But heavy use of these products may damage the kidneys, a fact that far outweighs the benefits of preventing osteoporosis. (Other medication is available to prevent this condition.) We therefore believe that high doses of antacids containing calcium should not be used routinely, except under the careful supervision of a physician.

Magnesium (Maalox, Mylanta, milk of magnesia, Camalox, Riopan, Gelusil)

Magnesium hydroxide is a compound found in virtually all noncalcium antacids. The compound causes diarrhea and is therefore the ingredient found in many laxatives. To counteract this effect, most magnesium-based antacids are mixed with aluminum-containing compounds. These medications have few side effects when used for a short time, but like calcium, magnesium can cause kidney stones and (no different from other antacids) be particularly dangerous in people with other kidney problems.

Aluminum (Rolaids, AlternaGEL, Amphojel)

Aluminum-containing antacids are most frequently used in combination with magnesium because aluminum alone causes constipation. Used over prolonged periods, at high doses, the chemical may also deplete the body of certain minerals (such as calcium and fluoride) that help prevent bone problems. Once again those with kidney problems are particularly at risk of this side effect.

One fear about these compounds that appears to have been put to rest is the link between aluminum and Alzheimer's disease. Scientific research has confirmed that these aluminum-based compounds are safe and effective for most people when taken in moderate doses.

Simethicone

Many antacids contain an ingredient called simethicone that reduces excess gas in the stomach and intestines. It is known as a "defoaming" agent that breaks up gas bubbles and hastens their elimination from the body. Although occasionally used alone in people with "gas problems," simethicone is more commonly included in antacid preparations such as Maalox, Mylanta, Riopan, Gelusil, and Di-Gel.

Alginic Acid (Gaviscon)

Gaviscon is not an antacid. Alginic acid creates a foam in the body like a bubble bath. This foam forms a barrier between the stomach and the esophagus. Therefore, even if the stomach acid is not neutralized, it theoretically cannot get to the part of the body where it can do the most damage. Scientific experiments confirm that Gaviscon gives about the same symptomatic relief as antacids. It has very few side effects.

To review, the principal active ingredients found in antacids are sodium bicarbonate, calcium, magnesium, aluminum, alginic acid, and simethicone—either alone or in combination. All the other ingredients you see on the packages are "inactive"; that means they affect not how the compounds work but how they look or taste.

Thus we see food colorings, sweeteners, dyes, and such flavorings as mint, cherry, and lemon. Be cautious of the mint taste. Many of my patients tell me that mint flavoring will initially make their heartburn worse before producing relief.

One other compound people frequently take for stomach problems is Pepto-Bismol. Some of my patients "can't live" without this comforting pink bottle because it seems almost immediately to help whatever is bothering them. The active ingredient in this liquid is bismuth, which has been shown to help heal stomach ulcers. Bismuth also soothes upset stomachs and relieves cramps and diarrhea. The confusion about the use of this medicine is related to the general confusion about terms used to describe stomach problems. Many people who use the term "indigestion" in the broadest sense are not referring to "heartburn" or reflux disease. These are the people who find Pepto-Bismol beneficial. But in true heartburn, where our goal is to neutralize stomach acid, Pepto-Bismol, like Alka-Seltzer, may be *harmful* because of its composition. Pepto-Bismol liquid does contain magnesium and aluminum, which make your stomach acid harmless, but it also contains an aspirinlike substance (subsalicylic acid) that can aggravate heartburn and may eventually cause other general stomach problems to become worse. Therefore, we recommend that this product, like Alka-Seltzer, be used with caution.

Let's summarize some important points. All the antacids on your supermarket shelf are relatively safe, and all will to some degree reduce the potency of the acid in your system and relieve your symptoms. *None* of the antacids is safe when used at high doses over a prolonged period of time. Some antacids present more danger than others to people with certain diseases or conditions, and certain combinations of antacid products should be avoided altogether:

- People with high blood pressure or on salt-restricted diets should avoid compounds containing sodium or sodium bicarbonate.
- People prone to constipation should avoid aluminum- and calcium-containing antacids, and those prone to diarrhea should be careful of magnesium-containing compounds.
- Anyone with kidney problems should be cautious about *all* antacids.

If you are taking *any* medication, you should talk to your doctor before taking antacids. Antacids can block the absorption of many compounds, most significantly the antibiotic tetracycline, isoniazid (a drug for tuberculosis), and iron.

Many of my patients don't seem to realize that antacids are classified as *medicines*. My colleagues and I have noted that people who frequently use antacids do not tell their doctors that they are using medication. In fact, they may tell us that they are in "perfect health." But perfect health is not a burning chest and incapacitating pain. Perfect health does not require taking medicine seven or eight times a day for years.

If antacids are not appropriate for many people, let's get an idea of whom they are useful for and how they can best be taken. Ironically, the people who are prime candidates for antacids never come to see me. These are the people who experience heartburn once or twice a month. While they may have pain on these occasions, it does not last long enough to compel the sufferers to see a doctor, and it does not interfere with daily routines. For these people, antacids are ideal.

My uncle Harry falls into this category. He gets heartburn only when he eats foods like chicken paprikash or spaghetti with spicy marinara sauce. When I tell him the best way to treat his heartburn is to avoid these foods, he lectures me about the pleasures and pitfalls of life. I will simply say that my uncle knows the price his body pays for eating his favorite foods and takes an antacid at the first hint of heartburn.

In these people—and there are many millions—an antacid provides safe, fast, and very effective relief. As for choosing the right antacid for you, that depends on your overall medical condition and the potency of the tablet or liquid.

Remember that jar of hydrochloric acid in my laboratory? If I want to neutralize the acid, I can add varying amounts of alkali (sodium bicarbonate, calcium, magnesium, or aluminum). And I can add various combinations. How effectively the compounds neutralize acid is known, unsurprisingly, as the acid-neutralizing capacity (ANC). Antacids are tested for ANC and rated on a numerical scale.

The ANC of antacids varies widely. The most potent liquid antacids, consequently the ones recommended most by gastroenterologists, are Maalox Plus, Mylanta II, and Riopan Plus 2. The least potent products in terms of neutralizing capacity are Amphojel and Di-Gel. You don't get a more powerful product by paying more money for it. Riopan Plus 2 is *less* expensive than Gelusil, despite the fact that Gelusil is less than half as powerful.

Liquid antacids have an advantage over tablets because they work faster. But patients often prefer the convenience of tablets.

The most potent brand-name tablets are Riopan Plus 2, Maalox TC, and Gelusil II. Some tablets, such as Titrilac and Tums, are very weak. As with liquid antacids, the price does not necessarily correlate with the potency. Further complicating matters is that manufacturers change the formulations, prices, and strengths of their antacids.

The least expensive way to purchase antacids is to buy a generic product from your drugstore. Because none of the ingredients in an antacid can be patented, any company can manufacture its own version.

We recommend any generic medication similar to Maalox Plus, Mylanta, Riopan, or Gelusil. Each of these drugs contains magnesium, aluminum, and simethicone. You can save yourself many dollars by simply asking your pharmacist for a generic version of these products.

We have already pointed out that most people use antacids incorrectly. The package instructions do a good job of instructing people not to take too much of the drug, but they do a terrible job of telling people how to use it. Many patients who come to see me believe they need a stronger medication than antacid. Some do. But others have been taking a dose of an antacid that is not high enough or taking their medicine at the wrong time.

Most antacid instructions present a fixed schedule for taking the product. By a "fixed schedule," we mean medication at regular intervals during the day (for example, two tablets in the morning, two in the afternoon, and two before going to bed). Fixed schedule medication is of benefit for treating an infection because an infection is a continuous process in the body, but antacids are recommended only for *episodic* heartburn, which by its nature is not a continuous process. Therefore, taking an antacid on a regular schedule is commonly a waste of time and money and needlessly exposes you to possible side effects. The appropriate time to take an antacid is when you feel symptoms or *as needed*.

Two other points are also important to remember. Antacids are *short-acting,* so they won't do you much good if your goal is to get a good night's sleep. Taking two tablets before going to bed may help for a few hours if that bedtime is some hours after eating, but you'll wake up in misery. Secondly, taking liquid antacids on an empty stomach may be less effective since they may quickly pass into the intestine; taking them one to two hours after eating often provides better symptomatic relief.

Odd as it may seem, many people take too *low* a dose of antacids. During an episodic attack heartburn can require a good deal of antacid to work properly, much more than the dosage stated on the bottle. You are dealing with surging hydrochloric acid here! *So cooperate with your physician to find the level of medication that is effective for you*. And keep in mind that you want to maintain this amount only when you have active heartburn symptoms. Don't gulp tablets all day or keep swigging from the antacid bottle.

If you are having active symptoms all the time and find yourself taking antacids continuously to get relief, you should see a physician. Your body is probably unable to cope with the flow of acid. Instead of needing an agent to neutralize it, you need medication to turn it off. (Think of an overflowing sink. If the tap is slightly open and water is spilling onto the floor, you can use a mop to wipe up the excess. But if the tap is wide open, all your mopping won't keep up with the spreading puddle.)

What is most amazing to me about antacid users is that instead of getting help turning off the faucet, they increase their mopping to a frantic pace. Many don't even realize what they are doing.

If your heartburn is keeping you up at night, if you associate food with misery, if antacids are causing you side effects, and if you find yourself constantly taking more and more of them, it's time to get medical help.

Antacids will not help those people with more serious reflux disease: those with chronic wheezing and cough, asthma, hoarseness, and irritations or ulcerations to any part of the esophagus or throat. Fortunately we no longer must rely on chemicals that have been around for thousands of years. In 1964 scientists in a British laboratory finally began to investigate how the body could decrease the flow of stomach acid. The answer eventually led many patients to lead a normal life and ushered in a new era in medical therapy.

4

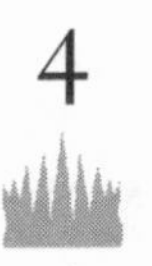

ACID DISEASE

Cause and Cure

> The mass of men lead lives of quiet desperation. What is called resignation is confirmed desperation.
>
> —*Henry David Thoreau,* Walden, or Life in the Woods, *1854*

When I was in college in the late 1960s, I gradually became aware that one of my best friends suffered from bouts of "severe indigestion." At first Scott didn't tell anyone because he felt "embarrassed and a little bit ashamed." But as his condition became worse, Scott found it impossible to hide his ailment. He began to make almost daily visits to the university clinic and was quickly put on a medical regimen of soft, bland food and antacids. In addition, he was tested for various stomach and intestinal disorders, but the tests revealed no physical problems. It wasn't until two decades later that my friend confided the rest of the story.

Scott was referred to a psychiatrist, who decided that

his young patient was "nervous and depressed" and needed a mild tranquilizer (Valium) and psychotherapy. Unfortunately the antacids, diet, psychological counseling, and Valium did not solve the problem. In fact, the illness became worse. While all his friends were having snacks at a diner famous for its Cokes, burgers, and fries (not to mention its greasy walls), Scott was sitting alone in the dorm cafeteria, taking sips from a large glass of milk. Severe heartburn has never improved anyone's social life, nor can it be called an uplifting experience, a fact that may account for its close association with the psychiatric profession.

It was on a freezing afternoon just after the midseason break that Scott's roommate called with bad news. Our friend's condition had worsened to the point that he was completely unable to eat and needed emergency treatment. The next day, when I went to visit Scott in the hospital, I was stunned. He was lying in bed, pale and confused, connected to tubes and bottles, staring glumly out the window. His voice was hoarse, and he spoke in a worried whisper. The hospital staff had discovered that Scott's esophagus was severely ulcerated and in danger of becoming blocked from scar tissue.

Therapy would consist of complete bed rest, liquid antacids, and feeding through tubes. If that didn't work, Scott would have to undergo a complicated operation that the doctors thought *might* help his condition. (The surgical failure rate was believed to be about 30 percent. The failure rate with medicine was estimated to be 80 percent.) In sum, Scott's illness was considered a *very* difficult management problem, and he was informed that he might have chronic and debilitating pain for the rest of his life.

Not a very pleasant prospect for a young man of twenty growing up in 1971.

I include this experience of my friend to illustrate how little progress had been made in the treatment of acid reflux since its recognition. In some ways matters had even gotten *worse* for reflux disease sufferers, because so much confusion, controversy, and disagreement surrounded the illness. As a result, patients were misdiagnosed or not diagnosed at all, given useless or harmful drugs, or branded as psychologically unstable. Some underwent surgery for essentially the wrong disease. Even now, when I see some of the patients in my office, I wonder just how much, if anything, has changed.

Medical science can at times be compared with an elaborate game of connect the dots, in which we try to follow a trail to the point of origin of a disease. Once we have found the point of origin, we at least know where to begin our search for a cure. Sometimes the trail is logical: Point a leads to point b, which leads to point c. A *pain* in an area near the stomach turns out to be caused by an *irritation* in the stomach, which is caused by a *substance* in the stomach. Such is the case with either a stomach or duodenal ulcer. A duodenal ulcer (which many people think of as a stomach ulcer) is an illness that involves a part of the small intestine just under the stomach. It is not a hard ailment to diagnose initially. A doctor presses down on the body, and the patient's pain usually increases.

By the early part of the twentieth century physicians using the new miracle device known as the X-ray machine and a liquid coating could peer inside the stomach and actually "see" an outline of stomach and duodenal ulcers. Thus, because of the obvious symptoms of abdominal pain and the rapid means of making a firm diagnosis, these forms of ulcers became well known to both physicians and the public.

Detecting and documenting ulcers and irritations of

the esophagus, as well as many other common manifestations of acid reflux has proved far more complicated, and many controversies remain today. It was not until the development of fiber optics and miniature television chips in the 1970s and 1980s that we could easily and safely examine the upper part of the digestive tract in close detail.

Making matters more complicated is the fact that reflux disease is the Great Masquerader and its symptoms may not make sense in terms of the actual source of the pain. Patients who later proved to have acid reflux complained of shortness of breath, wheezing, sour taste in the mouth, chest pain, loss of voice, back problems, dental problems, sore throats, colds, fatigue—you name it. The only common link was patient distress. Oftentimes even examination with the most sophisticated diagnostic tools failed to turn up the source of the problem.

Little wonder, then, that the road to relief of acid reflux has been twisting, misleading, and difficult. And no wonder that you or one of your friends or family members still suffer. What follows is a road map to the first real breakthroughs. It's actually a mystery tour that began in the 1800s and led more than a century later to two dramatic advances in the history of medicine.

By the nineteenth century heartburn had long been identified and physicians were aware that certain chemicals—antacids—could relieve the pain of the ailment. Despite this therapy, the condition remained widespread enough to be characterized as "America's national disease." Furthermore, no one yet realized that heartburn could be a symptom of a very serious physical condition.

Interestingly, at just about the time that Dr. Beaumont was learning about the effects of hydrochloric acid in the stomach, German researchers had identified a mysterious, heretofore unknown ailment that showed up during the autopsies of certain corpses: *ulcus oesophagi simplex,* ulcer of the esophagus.

Many of the people who were found to have had this disease were afflicted by a wide variety of other ailments. However, some had *no* known disorders, nor had they presented symptoms during their lifetime. The ulcers in the esophagus appeared to resemble those found in or near the stomach or intestine. Under the microscope scientists could clearly see tiny erosions or sores. But while Beaumont and others demonstrated the corrosive power of stomach acid and thus could identify the cause of the ulcers in that part of the body, no one was sure what was causing the ulcers in the esophagus. To add to the mystery, the stomachs of many people with esophageal ulcers were perfectly normal.

Scientists debated the medical condition for years and speculated that esophageal ulcers were the result of cancer, infections, tuberculosis, syphilis, even mental hysteria. At the turn of the twentieth century an American doctor named Wilder Tileston suggested that the strange illness was "more common than suspected," that it was not easy to diagnose, and that patients were at high risk. He guessed that the ailment might have some relationship to stomach acid but was unable to offer any proof. The cure he suggested was bismuth (the substance in Pepto-Bismol). If that didn't work (and there is no reason to think that it did), patients had to be fed directly into the body with a tube.

It never occurred to Tileston to treat this malady of the esophagus with antacids. By contrast, the cause and initial therapy of stomach and duodenal ulcer were beginning to be understood by the twentieth century, and the term "ulcer" became firmly associated in the mind of physicians and the public with a "stomach problem." In the decades after Tileston, some researchers began to suspect that ulcer of the esophagus and ulcer of the stomach and duodenum were part of the same disease. Crude devices, known as gastroscopes, made it possible to examine patients with erosions of the esophagus, and these sores looked suspiciously like stomach ulcers. Thus began the confusion that remains to this day. While the two ailments share certain characteristics (both are in part related to the corrosive effects of stomach acid), they are two distinct illnesses.

A well-respected consumer magazine that reviewed antacids in 1994 warned people they might have something more serious than heartburn—"an ulcer"—but the cautionary article referred only to ulcers of the stomach and intestine and never mentioned the more likely possibility of irritation or ulcer of the esophagus. Nor did the article mention the relationship of heartburn and acid reflux to asthma or hoarseness. No wonder reflux disease, heartburn, and the surrounding complications remain so poorly diagnosed and treated!

And no wonder I am sometimes the ninth or tenth doctor my patients come to see.

A leap forward in our understanding of reflux disease was made in 1936 by a New York physician named Asher Winkelstein, who at last clearly identified a condition he called "Peptic Esophagitis." He stated that the disease was chronic, was associated with heartburn, and was caused by the irritation of hydrochloric acid in stomach juices. He also speculated about the role of the sphincter (the valve between the esophagus and stomach) in this condition, but his real contribution was to make heartburn "respectable." At last it was linked with something harmful occurring in the body, something that physicians could actually see. Winkelstein still wondered whether a strong psychological factor was involved, but gone was any mention that the ailment was brought on by French novels. More important, because heartburn, injury to the esophagus, and stomach acid were now seen to be related, a therapy could at last be proposed.

Unfortunately it not only turned out to be the wrong therapy but made patients sicker.

By the 1930s it was known that certain drugs could limit the production of stomach acid. Scientists were beginning to unravel the mystery of how acid was made and how chemicals could be used to halt it. One such chemical was atropine, which was the first medication added to Dr. Sippy's basic regimen for quieting acid and helping stomach and duodenal ulcer patients. But atropine affects many different parts of the body (in addition to the stomach) and causes a number of serious side effects, including dryness of mouth and urinary, heart, and vision problems. Hardly the ideal drug for a patient already plagued by a crippling sickness!

Or as one of my professors in medical school put it, "Here we have a half-starved, hospitalized patient eating mush and milk, crammed full of antacids, and now he's finally given a drug, atropine, that makes him see double." (The story is often told of one woman on this early therapy who grew so disgusted that still wearing her gown, she ran out of the hospital, walked into a nearby diner, and consumed a full meal of turkey, potatoes, and stuffing. When the orderlies finally caught up with her, she told them she "would rather die on a full stomach than live in grief on an empty one.")

But as miserable as the regimen was for stomach and duodenal ulcer patients, it was sheer agony for those with severe heartburn caused by inflammation of the esophagus. Winkelstein's patients were treated with olive oil before meals, milk, and soft cereal—antacids and atropine. Olive oil was thought to coat and protect the stomach, the calcium in milk was thought to neutralize acid, and soft, bland cereal was thought to be nonirritating. Antacids and atropine were added to neutralize acid further and slow its production. But what the regimen really did was very different, especially to the patient with acid reflux. Milk (which contained fat and calcium) at first calmed the acid, then increased it; antacids caused either diarrhea or constipation; and atropine (the new wonder drug) was found later to make it *easier* for stomach acid to flow up to the esophagus.

Heartburn sufferers would probably have been better off on Galen's theriac of the first century or Paracelsus's "amalgam" of the sixteenth.

Perhaps because no effective medical therapy proved itself for severe heartburn or inflammation and ulcer of the esophagus, doctors refocused their search for a cure on correcting what they believed to be the basic structural problem in the body. This was a hiatus hernia, which simply referred to an extension of the stomach above the diaphragm. It was believed that when this hiatus hernia "slid" from its normal position, reflux disease and its symptoms were the result. In the 1940s and 1950s this term, "sliding hiatal hernia" or "symptomatic hiatus hernia," was used interchangeably with terms referring to reflux disease, and the confusion still exists among many of my older patients.

The hiatal hernia was repaired by means of an operation, but not many people with reflux disease got better. As it turned out, a hiatal hernia and acid reflux may be linked, but such occurrence is often coincidental. A study completed in 1968 indicated that of all people with hiatal hernias, only 24 percent had esophagitis, and of patients with esophagitis, only 45 percent had hiatal hernias. So once again reflux disease sufferers who underwent the hiatal hernia operation were given an inappropriate treatment. In this same period stomach ulcer patients were also treated surgically, either with a procedure that cut the nerves that stimulated acid secretion or by removal of part or all of the stomach itself. Stomach ulcer patients were at least getting therapy that could alleviate their condition. The hiatal hernia operation as a remedy for acid reflux was largely useless and is currently no longer an option.

By the sixties and seventies other operations more directly linked to reflux disease had been developed. These procedures tighten the sphincter and theoretically thus prevent the flow of acid into the esophagus. They are very tricky procedures, and their success depends largely on the skill of the surgeon. As we shall see in chapter 9, there is still debate about how effective the procedures are. In any case they are too complex and sometimes too risky to help any but the most severely afflicted patients.

Additionally, just as some people are sensitive or prone to the side effects of medication, so others cannot easily tolerate surgery. They may have illnesses that would make all but the most critical operation unwise, or frankly, they may have unwillingness or fear. Such was the case with my college friend Scott, who in 1972 was taking antacids eight times a day for his acid reflux. Scott knew very little about the discouraging history of therapy for his condition. But he was a philosophy major and extremely bright, and one day (when he was in the hospital for intravenous feeding), he said to me, "You know, Mike, I don't think these people have any idea what's the matter with me." Scott was wrong; they had *many, many* ideas, but what they lacked was a good therapy.

In 1964 a brilliant scientist named James Black joined a group of researchers in the British laboratories of a Philadelphia-based pharmaceutical company, Smith Kline & French. Black was already famous for inventing a class of medications still widely used. These drugs, the beta-blockers (Inderal, Lopressor, Tenormin, Corgard), revolutionized the treatment of high blood pressure and other heart problems. Dr. Black hoped he could revolutionize the treatment of stomach and duodenal ulcer disease by using the same formula he had devised for developing the beta-blockers: Identify the chemical that causes the problem (in this case stomach acid production); then find another chemical that blocks the action of this stimulating agent.

Black thought the search would take a few years. But it took more than a decade and involved the near demise of Smith Kline & French, numerous corporate threats to cut off funds, years of incorrect leads, the production of numerous toxic substances—and the dedication of a fanatic staff—before Black's goal was realized.

It all involved the search for a blocker of the chemical "histamine" that had long been suspected as a cause of stomach acid production. Histamine is a familiar chemical because it causes most of our allergy problems and many of the miseries of the common cold. Persons suffering from hay fever have taken an "*anti*histamine" (like Benadryl) because it is the ingredient found in practically every cold remedy on the drugstore shelf. (It doesn't cure colds, but it does "dry up" nasal passages. More important, it makes you drowsy so that you fall asleep.) Your allergy medicine works because it "blocks" the effect of histamine and therefore prevents sneezing attacks, headaches, rashes, and other symptoms of colds and allergies.

It had long been thought that a compound linked to histamine or perhaps a different form of histamine itself caused the stomach to make more acid. Black wondered: What if the effects of *this* compound could be blocked? Would it prevent stomach ulcers the way allergy medicine prevented runny nose and hives? Proving this theory was a more difficult task than anyone could imagine. Part of the problem was to determine first *if* it was even possible to create a new form of histamine blocker, one that blocked only acid production, without causing undesirable side effects. The subsequent obstacles to overcome would then be to create a drug and test its effects in living organisms.

Black's teammates faced an enormous task even before any kind of medication could be developed, let alone tested. Gradually they moved forward, first confirming that the second form of histamine blocker could be created, then designing models to test how it might work, and finally experimenting on compounds they hoped would shut off stomach acid.

By 1969 the research team had investigated more than seven hundred compounds that decreased acid flow. None of these was successful, and many were toxic. Corporate pressure on Black's team was intense, and finances were depleted. The urgency to show results and create a useful medicine was so crushing that researchers worked nights by candlelight during a coal miners' strike when electricity was cut off.

Finally there seemed a breakthrough with the development of a more sophisticated method to measure the effectiveness of compounds in shutting off stomach acid. An experiment was designed to test a new medicine in the stomach of a dog. The dog was fed a diet that caused it to produce a large amount of acid; then the new drug was introduced. "It was like magic," Dr. Michael Parsons, a member of the team, recalled. "Suddenly all the acid in the dog's stomach just disappeared."

The surprise was that the new medicine seemed to be blocking much more acid than the researchers ever hoped it would. From the modest goal of unraveling and understanding histamine, Black's team seemed to have found a compound that blocked *all* the chemical messengers in the body that stimulated stomach acid.

"No one expected this," Dr. Parsons said. "It not only helped us find a cure but opened a whole window on how stomach acid worked."

That night the team went to a local pub in the rolling hills around Hertfordshire and had a very late celebration. In 1971 research director Bill Duncan became the first human to swallow a drug that prevented histamine from stimulating stomach acid. "I'm not sure what any of us thought would happen," Duncan recalled. Later corporate headquarters in Philadelphia inquired if Duncan "had checked with corporate personnel about his life insurance."

Unfortunately the compound proved to cause toxic side effects related to bone marrow depletion. Seven years of concentrated effort had yielded a harmful compound, and many experts throughout the world remained highly skeptical of Dr. Black's work. At a symposium at Johns Hopkins Hospital in 1973 a leading gastroenterologist stated that chemicals that blocked the acid-stimulating effects of histamine were "inherently toxic."

There were a number of reasons for this concern. First, production of acid has always been considered a normal function of the stomach, and doctors thought that when this normal function was blocked, harmful effects could result. Stomach acid was believed to play an important role in preventing the growth of certain forms of bacteria in the digestive tract, and it was speculated that this excess bacteria could convert nitrates and nitrites (preservatives found in many foods) into chemicals (nitrosamines) known to be linked to cancer. But it has since been determined that this concern is merely theoretical, and there has actually been a marked *decrease* in the rate of cancer of the stomach in the United States and other Western nations.

Secondly, researchers discovered that numerous people who produced no stomach acid whatsoever led completely normal lives. (This fact comes as a considerable surprise to many of my patients.) Millions of people with no stomach acid can digest food perfectly well. So the next question is: If we can live without it, why does the body make stomach acid in the first place? The answer may lie in the fact that human beings did not always eat cooked, relatively hygienic foods. Stomach acid production among animals serves a valuable function in killing the bacteria ingested from eating raw meat and other contaminated substances.

Those of us who do not eat bacteria-ridden food should have no concern, therefore, about taking medication that decreases our stomach acid production. Like many functions in the body, our acid-producing system works as a backup. We don't really need it, but it's helpful to have around in case other systems fail.

In 1971, however, safety concerns about stomach acid–blocking drugs were an important issue. It was only after Black's team tested another drug it was developing called Tagamet that a safe acid blocker came into general use. It was first tried in actual medical practice on a severely ill patient who had had a very bad reaction to the first histamine or H2 blocker. The decision to proceed was crucial, a last fling of the dice. If the drug worked, the program would continue. If it didn't, it is likely that one of the most promising forms of therapy in the twentieth century would have been abandoned.

Tagamet did work. It was now more than seven years after James Black had speculated about what caused duodenal and stomach ulcers, and at last scientists had a compound that appeared both effective and safe. In 1976 Tagament was introduced for human use in Britain, and in the next two years it was approved throughout the world.

For the first time a simple tablet could finally accomplish what elixirs, theriac, seltzer, voodoo spells, fasts, numerology, astrology, milk, oatmeal, antacids, burned paper, and atropine could not: safely and effectively decrease the flow of stomach acid and prevent it from eating away the body's tissues. For his achievements, James Black was knighted and received the Nobel Prize in medicine.

What happened next is a story partly of medicine, partly of epidemiology, and partly of astonishment because Tagamet's success greatly surpassed the expectations of even its most impassioned boosters. In just one year it became the most widely prescribed drug in the world. The reason now seems simple. No one appreciated the number of people who were affected by acid reflux or the fact that, to echo Thoreau, they were leading lives of quiet desperation. That desperation turned highly vocal.

Inspired by front-page headlines about a miracle ulcer cure, patients with every conceivable stomach condition raced into doctors' offices to demand the new medication. For many, including those with the milder forms of heartburn, it worked like a charm.

Other pharmaceutical manufacturers were quick to take advantage of Tagamet's popularity, and three other drugs that blocked the effects of histamine (H2 blockers) were introduced—Zantac, Pepcid, and Axid—each becoming an enormous success. Zantac is the largest-selling medication in the world today and currently earns its manufacturer more money every year than the entire annual revenue of Smith Kline & French before the introduction of Tagamet.

Considering the remarkable number of people who have taken these medications for so many years, we can confidently say that the early safety worries did not pan out. H2 blockers have very few side effects and can be safely taken for long periods. In many countries, including the United States, Tagamet and Pepcid can now be purchased without a doctor's prescription and used "as needed" by the patient. I am certain that Zantac and Axid too will be approved soon for over-the-counter use.

Not even Sir James Black himself could have predicted the virtual industry that would arise from the discovery of a new form of antihistamine.

The first and most immediate effect of Tagamet's approval and the subsequent use of other H2 blockers was to lower dramatically the rate for surgery and hospital admissions for stomach and duodenal ulcers. One of the most significant declines was documented at the Mayo Clinic in Rochester, Minnesota. The number of operations decreased from forty-nine per hundred thousand patients to six per hundred thousand in the early 1980s. The rate of hospital admissions for milder forms of duodenal ulcer declined about 50 percent in the same time period.

The H2 blockers also had a profound effect on the general practice of medicine. The family doctor could now treat the average stomach or duodenal ulcer patient without resorting to drastic diets, massive doses of antacids, or hospitalization and surgery. And the focus of gastroenterologists like me returned once again to medicine, rather than surgery. (Directors of surgical training programs throughout the United States began to complain that they were unable to teach medical students and residents the necessary operations that were historically used to treat duodenal ulcers.)

I vividly recall from my internship the story of a patient named Pete. He had a history of duodenal ulcers dating back to his teenage years, with bout after bout of severe abdominal pain. Two months after he was married, he developed a bleeding duodenal ulcer so serious that it required an operation to cut the nerves to the stomach that stimulate acid. After this procedure Pete did well, much to the relief of the hospital staff, Pete's wife, and, of course, Pete himself.

Pete was an extremely bright and insightful young man, but like many people who suffer from stomach ailments, he tended to blame both himself and whatever was going on in his life for his condition. "No, Pete," I told him for two years, "it was not your wife who gave you an ulcer; it was hydrochloric acid."

"You don't know my wife," he protested.

"I know you, Pete," I said, "and I know your stomach."

In fact, despite a fairly calm and peaceful homelife, two years after the first operation, Pete suddenly developed the same symptoms that had preceded his initial hospital stay. A leading gastroenterologist at our medical center (a physician in his late fifties) recommended that Pete undergo another operation, this time a more drastic and potentially dangerous procedure to remove the lower portion of his stomach. Pete's personal physician vetoed the idea (a risky thing to do with stomach ulcer patients in the late seventies). He had read about the work of James Black and the increasing reports of success with the new acid-suppressing medication.

Pete was given the drug immediately after it was released in the United States and never again suffered abdominal pain or bleeding.

But what about my friend Scott? The patient with heartburn and esophagitis? Scott was not initially given Tagamet for his condition, nor were many others like him. The Food and Drug Administration of the United States, and many other regulatory agencies throughout the world, did not give approval for Tagamet's use for either heartburn or many other illnesses related to stomach acid production. This was not a case of uncaring regulatory agencies. It was a case of science being unable to show (as it had so clearly and dramatically with stomach and duodenal ulcers) that the medication worked.

The good news for Scott was that he made a sufficient recovery from his heartburn to avoid an operation. The bad news was that his misery continued. Eventually he was put on a treatment regime of Tagamet and antacids. It did some good ("My life went from being total hell to half hell"), but not enough to allow him a normal life or, more ominously, to heal the erosions in his esophagus.

The difference between what happened with Pete, who made a complete recovery on Tagamet, and Scott, who barely responded, is very important for you to understand. As we have emphasized a number of times, *duodenal and stomach ulcers are not the same illnesses as esophageal ulcers, irritations, heartburn, and other conditions caused by the reflux of stomach acid. They may appear the same; they may even have very similar symptoms. But they are not the same ailment and cannot be treated the same way*. It was because researchers made this mistake in the early 1980s, when they first attempted to prove that Tagamet would work on reflux disease, that the drug showed poor results on this condition. You can't treat GERD the same way as you treat stomach or duodenal ulcer. By 1994 science had established this fact beyond a reasonable doubt. But medicine has been slow to change, and as a result, millions of patients remain in unnecessary pain and at unnecessary risk.

Let's go back to the late 1970s to understand the problem more fully. When Tagamet was first studied, it was tested at very high doses. Even when it first came on the market, it was thought that because the effect of the drug was not long-lasting, it would have to be given to duodenal ulcer patients four times a day. However, as doctors developed a better understanding of the effects of Tagamet and how stomach and duodenal ulcers were formed, they found that *much* lower doses would effectively eliminate and control most cases. The established therapy (which worked on more than 80 percent of patients) became one dose of Tagamet taken a few hours after dinner. The reason: In stomach and duodenal ulcer patients, a large proportion of the body's acid is produced after the last meal of the day and in the middle of the night. Therefore, despite the fact that Tagamet did not work for a long period, one dose taken in the evening controlled acid during the critical periods of acid production. After the duodenal ulcer healed, doctors could prescribe an even lower dose to keep patients from a relapse.

But while this daily dose of Tagamet proved a miracle for patients with stomach and duodenal ulcers, it did not prove very effective for patients like Scott with heartburn *and* esophagitis. Nor did the drug improve the condition of many people with more severe forms of heartburn or those with asthma, hoarseness, or chest pain.

One reason is that acid reflux is a chronic illness. As all people who pop antacids know, it flares up constantly. Except in mild forms, it cannot be treated for a short time because stomach acid is almost always bubbling up into the esophagus. In many reflux patients, acid must be tamed all the time. Therefore, taking an H2 blocker once a day will not control the disease. It is a case of a pill that does not work for very long being used to treat an illness that occurs around the clock.

In addition, because acid reflux is a chronic illness that often maintains the same level of severity, many patients require the same dose of medicine all the time. It is not a question of getting rid of a disease, then preventing it from coming back, as with stomach or duodenal ulcer.

Another problem with a short-acting drug is that many parts of the body that are affected by the reflux of stomach acid are extremely sensitive. Even a small amount of hydrochloric acid will prevent the esophagus or larynx from healing. Like the special flask in my laboratory, the stomach was designed to house acid; the esophagus was not.

Finally, the H2 blockers take from thirty to sixty minutes to work, and if you've ever experienced piercing heartburn, you know that even a half hour can seem a lifetime.

In fact, many heartburn patients who tried the H2 blockers in their original low dose went *back* to antacids. Relief was faster and more dependable. I call this the pizza principle. Most people take medication *after* pain, not before it happens. So they order pizza, *then* take their Tagamet or Zantac. Misery continues, and the patient (along with his or her doctor) concludes that the drug doesn't work for heartburn. Bear in mind that the H2 blocker does not neutralize acid; it decreases its production. Therefore, when you get an attack of heartburn, even if you take one of these drugs, reflux of acid continues for a while—and pain does not stop.

Think again of the overflowing sink. If water has overflowed, turning off the faucet would prevent more water from falling on the floor. However, it would not take care of the water that has already overflowed. You'd have to wait for this water to evaporate or drain or engage in a mop-up.

Gradually, as physicians became more confident with regard to the H2 blockers, gained practical experience, and actually saw how the drugs worked on patients, they learned that many people with acid reflux could be better helped by increasing the dose of these compounds and carefully regulating the time of day they were given.

A reflux patient with no significant complications can

generally be treated with an H2 antagonist in *two* daily doses. I usually recommend taking the medication between breakfast and lunch and one hour after dinner. By doing this, you are decreasing acid before it has "overflowed," thus controlling the problem before it starts.

But few general rules apply to heartburn. Acid reflux appears in so many forms that each person needs individual therapy. The best time to take your reflux medication can vary according to your eating schedule, your sleeping habits, the amount of exercise you receive, and, of course, the severity of your disease.

You may need one tablet twice a day or two tablets four times a day. There is no hard-and-fast rule. I had one patient whose doctor insisted he take his heartburn medication at night. The patient duly complied and felt miserable. But the doctor had read all the research and *knew* that the best time to take reflux medication was before going to bed. What the doctor never asked was when his patient slept! The man was a cabdriver who worked evenings to early morning, during which time he rarely ate. At about 4:00 A.M. the patient had a huge "breakfast" and went to sleep. Needless to say, he rarely had very pleasant dreams.

In sum, the H2 blockers—Tagamet, Zantac, Pepcid, and Axid—can work wonders on many with acid reflux, if and only if they are taken properly. Unfortunately no matter how much of these drugs are used, a significant number of people will *not* be helped. My friend Scott was one of them. His doctors raised the dose of his Zantac, Pepcid, Axid, and Tagamet (he tried them all) as high as modern medicine would allow, and still his symptoms remained.

But better news was ahead. As Sir James Black and his team were just concluding their research in England, another group in Sweden was developing a medication that would revolutionize the treatment of reflux disease in the same way that the H2 blockers revolutionized the treatment of stomach and duodenal ulcer.

This compound became known as Prilosec.

5

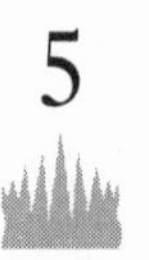

THE NEXT REVOLUTION

The belly is the reason why man does not mistake himself for a god.
—*Friedrich Nietzsche,* Beyond Good and Evil, *1886*

I became one of the first group of doctors in the United States to use this revolutionary drug. Prilosec had been prescribed in Europe for about two years, and I had eagerly read reports about it. However, like most physicians, I was somewhat skeptical about how well it really worked. By 1988 I had used Tagamet for more than a decade and could not imagine the practice of medicine without it. But more than one out of three of my reflux disease patients did not get relief, no matter how high a dosage of Tagamet or any of the H2 blockers I prescribed.

More alarmingly, I began to be concerned that among a significant number of my patients who had various degrees of irritation or ulcers of the esophagus, the H2 blockers were not effective. This surprised me and many of my colleagues. We naturally thought that if we had a medication that controlled stomach acid production, we could control acid-related illness. But because we never had a way of testing this idea, we really did not understand many basic facts about reflux disease.

Tagamet and its successors had a profound effect not only on therapy, but also on our *knowledge* of acid reflux. We confirmed that it was a distinct ailment, we learned more about its causes, we discovered new sets of symptoms, and we saw once again how difficult it was to treat. Perhaps not surprisingly to you, we also learned how widespread and debilitating heartburn was.

In order to overcome the limitations of the H2 blockers, I combined these medications with a variety of other drugs, some of which you may be taking. One, called Reglan, is a medication that improves digestion by moving food and acid more rapidly through the gastrointestinal tract and preventing it from moving back up. When combined with an H2 blocker, it eases symptoms of acid reflux but still cannot help the healing of the esophagus. Reglan is also limited by the fact that at least one of every five people cannot stand the side effects, the most common of which are fatigue and restlessness.

Another newer drug, somewhat similar to Reglan, although safer, more effective, and with fewer side effects is Propulsid. This drug improves digestion, primarily by helping the functioning of the sphincter, and is also effective in alleviating many of the symptoms of reflux disease. It is about as good as the H2 blockers in terms of healing the esophagus among patients with mild reflux disease, but it has limited effectiveness on patients with more severe forms of the illness. Propulsid has the further disadvantage of sometimes having to be taken at least two, three, or four times a day.

Finally, a drug known as Carafate has also been used for acid reflux. It works by coating the lining of the gastrointestinal tract and hence, at least theoretically, forming a barrier that prevents acid from damaging sensitive tissue. Unfortunately, despite the fact that this medicine has been available since the early 1980s, few good studies have tested its effectiveness in healing reflux disease.

In 1986 my friend Scott joined a large study to determine whether therapy with the then-approved medications or surgery that involved tightening the sphincter was superior. The medication group first received Zantac, antacids, and Reglan. If that did not work, patients were also given Carafate. Scott was in the medical group. By this time he considered himself something of an expert on acid reflux because of the number of drugs he had taken, the hospitals he had frequented, and the doctors he had seen.

Scott told me he did not mind the side effects of the drugs so much as the fact that he needed a portable alarm clock to make sure he was taking them all at the right time. He also used to keep a small diary to help him remember which hour to take which tablet.

The results of this study were reported in 1992 in the *New England Journal of Medicine* and showed that surgery was superior to medicine. But what the research really found was that neither drugs nor surgery were satisfactory for most patients and that the side effects of both kinds of treatments were numerous. This was particularly unfortunate because this clinical trial firmly and scientifically established that a sickness, now called gastroesophageal reflux disease (GERD), was chronic and required-long term treatment. Of course, given the fact that Scott had suffered with the ailment since his teenage years, he was not particularly surprised by these findings. Like so many others, he had more or less resigned himself to quiet desperation and assumed that pain was simply his lot in life.

As a specialist in a large teaching hospital I am often, regrettably, the physician of last resort. That is to say, patients come to see me after they have given up on everyone else. For this reason, I see all too many very sick people who are more inclined to take chances on new therapies because everything else has failed. Throughout the seventies and eighties I had tried combinations of drugs similar to those used in the *New England Journal* study but had achieved only limited success. Even if all the drugs worked for acid reflux (and they didn't), few patients were as diligent as Scott when it came to taking them.

As a general rule it is impractical to prescribe medication that has to be taken more than two or three times a day, every day, and ask a patient to stay the course.

However, we doctors simply had no choice. In 1985 the best we could do for our more severe heartburn patients was to try to give them drugs at least four times a day and hope for the best. So you can imagine how skeptical I was when I heard about a medication that could be taken *one* time a day, eliminate the symptoms of heartburn in virtually every patient, *and* heal the irritations and ulcers in the esophagus in more than 90 percent of cases! Furthermore, sufferers did not have to change their lifestyles, continue to take antacids, or alter their diets.

In effect, this new drug, Prilosec, promised to do even more for reflux and heartburn than what Tagamet had done for stomach and duodenal ulcers. Naturally I was both anxious and excited when I received special permission from the U.S. Food and Drug Administration to use Prilosec *before* it was approved in the United States. The FDA allows pharmaceutical companies to give small amounts of unapproved drugs for patients who show extraordinary need. This is called a "compassionate use" exception, and it is granted for only the sickest patients who have failed every approved course of therapy.* Such was the instance with one of my patients with a rare form of acid-related disease known as the Zollinger-Ellison syndrome.

This unusual illness was discovered at Ohio State University in 1955 by two surgeons who detected an ailment characterized by a huge output of stomach acid. This acid surge caused ulcerations so severe that no course of medical therapy could heal them. In fact, many of the original patients discovered with this disease died of terrible ulcer complications.

In the 1960s it became apparent that if the *entire* stomachs of such patients were removed, they would have a better chance of survival, but extension of life, much less better health, was by no means certain. After the discovery of the H2 blockers, we finally had an alternative to radical surgery. However, the medications had

*The Food and Drug Administration has eased these rules in recent years in the case of such potentially fatal illnesses as AIDS. However, it is generally true that obtaining any medication before FDA approval is difficult.

to be given in enormous doses, and the results were still unsure.

My first experience with Prilosec occurred with a woman named Joyce who came to see me with an uncontrolled form of Zollinger-Ellison syndrome. She was being treated with Zantac every four hours, around the clock—at a dose that was *twelve* times the usual level given for common stomach ulcer. Even with this enormous amount of medication, Joyce's health was in danger from the excess production of stomach acid. (Nor was her condition helped by the fact that she never slept through the night.)

After examining Joyce and realizing how serious the situation was, I requested Prilosec from the pharmaceutical manufacturer. The company and the FDA, recognizing my patient's precarious condition, granted the compassionate exception, and I soon received the new medication.

With Joyce's consent, I took her off her medical therapy of around-the-clock Zantac and replaced it with one large dose of Prilosec. It did not really seem possible to me that medicine given once a day would help a condition that had been considered fatal, but I crossed my fingers and gave Joyce precise instructions on how to reach me day or night if the medication did not work. The alternative to Prilosec was clear. If the medication did not work, Joyce would certainly have to undergo a difficult and potentially dangerous operation to remove her stomach.

Where did Prilosec come from and how was it developed? The story is as strange and twisting as the discovery of Tagamet. It could be said to have begun in 1946, when a group of hospital researchers found that a common local anesthetic called Xylocaine prevented the production of stomach acid. (Xylocaine is still widely used by dentists to numb pain.)

Nothing came of this observation until 1966, when a group of Swedish researchers, among them Dr. Lars Olbe, were assembled by Hässle Laboratories to see if they could find a compound that would stop acid production but not put people asleep. Like the team that worked with Sir James Black, these scientists were motivated by the fact that no effective medical treatment existed for stomach and duodenal ulcers. But while Black's team was attempting to unravel the mystery of histamine, a chemical that *indirectly* leads to the production of stomach acid, the Hässle group wanted to find a compound that blocked acid directly at the site where it was actually produced in the stomach.

Neither team knew of the other's efforts, although each group experienced the same frustration of continued failure. When British researchers announced the discovery of Tagamet in 1971, the Swedish group had managed to find only one promising new compound. Unfortunately what looked good in the laboratories did not work in humans. Six years of effort had produced little more than disappointment.

A chance observation sparked new interest. In 1972 the Swedes learned about a compound that had been developed to fight viral infections but coincidentally reduced stomach acid production. The pill turned out to be harmful when tested in animals, but the scientists thought they could alter the compound to eliminate the toxicity, while keeping its ability to diminish stomach acid.

It took two more years to develop such a medication and begin testing it. In 1974, just as Tagamet was in the last stages of human development, a drug named timoprazole was first being studied in animals. "We began to get enormously excited," recalls Dr. Enar Carlsson, who worked on the Prilosec team. "Dr. James Black had done a brilliant job of unraveling part of the mystery of acid secretion, but our team had gone a step further. We had finally developed a compound that seemed to work at the very spot where stomach acid was produced."

The scientists learned some very important facts. There is a pump within the stomach that produces acid, and in order for this "pump" to work, it needs to be stimulated by a number of chemicals, among them histamine. If you turn off the histamine, the pump will slow down and won't put out as much acid, but it will continue to allow acid to flow. The Swedish compound worked directly *inside* the pump, in effect enabling it to be shut off completely.

In fact, the concept of an "acid pump" in the stomach had also evolved in the United States, and some researchers were already attempting to find a compound similar to that of the Swedish group. One of these Americans, Dr. George Sachs, began a collaboration with the Swedes that eventually led to a new acid pump inhibitor and a greater understanding of the workings of the stomach.

But in 1977 timoprazole and a similar drug proved to have harmful effects in experimental animals, and research was halted. "The company had had enough at this point," Dr. Carlsson recalls. "We had been working for eleven years and had only a couple of toxic compounds to show for it." Just as Sir James's team had pleaded years before, so the Swedish scientists begged their company to let them continue. A quirk of fate intervened to help matters. A third related compound that had been developed named omeprazole (Prilosec) also seemed to cause harmful effects in the test animals. However, it turned out that the dogs had been affected not by this drug but through an inherited genetic problem. Research continued.

In 1979 a Danish physician named Simon Rune first tested the compound on a very sick human patient with Zollinger-Ellison syndrome. It looked as if thirteen years of intense research had finally paid off, for astonishingly, the patient's acid secretion was normalized in one *hour*.

The scientists decided to test Prilosec on a wider number of patients, and the results reported in 1982 were remarkable. However, as had happened with the Tagamet team, the Swedes faced a physician audience worried about the potential for harm. The development of Prilosec was therefore delayed for a year until issues regarding the drug's side effects in rats could be clarified. It was learned that certain abnormalities or "growths" appeared in the stomachs of rodents if they were given either Prilosec or high doses of H2 blockers over the entire life-spans of the rats. The Swedish and American coworkers concluded that the growths or cell clusters were therefore related not to Prilosec but to a chemical related to the suppression of acid. Most important, these abnormalities did not show up in any other nonrodent animals, and they have never appeared in humans after more than ten years of use.

Prilosec was first approved for public use in France in 1987. It had now been twenty-one years since the Hässle team had started its research, but it had finally accomplished the development of a safe and effective compound that could almost completely shut off stomach acid.

What happened next paralleled the reaction to Tagamet. It had been the goal of the Swedish scientists to find an agent to combat stomach and duodenal ulcers—certainly afflicting a sizable number of people—but the success of Prilosec went beyond every projection. "None of us realized how serious and widespread reflux disease was," Dr. Carlsson says, echoing the sentiment of Michael Parsons. But now that GERD could finally be treated and even severe heartburn controlled, doctors found that just as after the release of Tagamet, patients seemed to materialize right out of thin air.

Despite the fact that I had given careful instructions to my patient Joyce to phone me immediately if she had any problems with Prilosec, she never called.

Two weeks later she returned to my office looking happier and healthier than I had ever seen her, and I will never forget her first words. "I slept through the night," she said. "I actually slept through the night."

Using a sophisticated diagnostic tool, I measured the level of acid Joyce's body was making. It was normal.

Just to make sure, I measured it one more time, and the results were the same. I saw for myself what Swedish scientists had observed many years before: the action of a drug that could quickly and effectively normalized stomach acid.

I used the medication with three more patients before it was approved in the United States in 1989, each time with a successful outcome. Finally I was convinced. We now had a pill that could treat reflux disease as effectively as we could treat ulcers of the duodenum and stomach, and heartburn patients could now be quickly healed with a single tablet. In 1995 a second acid pump inhibitor similar to Prilosec, named Prevacid, was approved by the FDA for use in the United States.

Reflux disease is such a difficult illness to diagnose and may present with so many symptoms (or no symptoms at all) that physicians had no clear understanding of the usefulness of Prilosec. We knew that indigestion and heartburn were widespread; we knew that the histamine blockers worked for many people with acid reflux, but we did not know how many people had symptoms or physical damage that could not be controlled with the histamine blockers.

In a sense we had the same problem in 1989 that Wilder Tileston had had in 1905. Examining the esophagus is not something that is done during the average physical unless the patient complains of severe heartburn symptoms. And even then most doctors will try drug therapy to see if the patient gets better. It has been assumed that if the patient's symptoms improved, the underlying physical condition, if any, also improved. But we now know that is not necessarily the case. The symptoms of heartburn may be improved or totally eliminated by antacids, drugs like Propulsid, or even the histamine blockers. But the irritation in the esophagus remains.

Another factor that misled us about the number of people who would need a stronger acid-suppressing medication was that patients felt "better" on histamine blockers but did not feel truly normal. Patients were so happy that they were getting at least partial relief that they did not even expect complete relief.

Finally, at about the time that Prilosec was approved, we began to learn that a large number of people with acid reflux do not have the symptoms of heartburn as their *most* frequent complaint. As doctors used more sensitive diagnostic instruments and started prescribing higher doses of the histamine blockers to treat reflux disease, other symptoms and ailments began to disappear along with heartburn. These symptoms, which often appear in conjunction with acid reflux, include asthma, hoarseness, wheezing, and coughing, but it was not until we could use Prilosec that the association between these ailments and reflux disease could be confirmed.

No one could have foreseen that perhaps half the asthmatics in the United States (six million people) would respond to acid-suppressing therapy, millions more with hoarseness and loss of voice would be helped, and hundreds of thousands with severe chest pain (unrelated to heart disease) could get almost total relief.

Certainly I was surprised. As word about Prilosec spread in the medical community, I was deluged with patients, many of whom had long histories of vague and mysterious sicknesses. Family doctors who had either ignored or shrugged off their patients with heartburn and other forms of acid-related disease now started paying closer attention. Centuries-old medical theories about the relationship between stomach acid and various diseases such as asthma were finally being tested and verified. The great 1910 German medical dictum *Ohne sauren Magensaft, kein peptisches Geschwür*" ("No acid, no ulcer") could now be modified to "No acid, no heartburn." By studying the actions and effects of Prilosec, we are now making rapid progress toward understanding reflux disease, and we now recommend fewer and fewer patients for surgical procedures.

One of the first patients I saw after Prilosec approval was a gruff financial executive in his late fifties named Jack. In reviewing his history, I noted that Jack had suffered from heartburn nearly all his life. He was a walking textbook since he had tried every standard therapy (and quite a few others recommended by well-meaning family, friends, and even stockbrokers).

Like many older acid reflux patients, he was disillusioned with doctors and medicine in general since nothing had made him feel better and a good many therapies had made him feel worse. He had gotten some relief with Tagamet and later Zantac, but taking the tablets four times a day was "an impossible task." A dedicated and hardworking member of a large Boston firm, Jack would frequently be with a client or working on complex calculations and forget his medication. Needless to say, he paid dearly later.

A few weeks before Jack saw me, his physician had switched him to Prilosec and informed him that it would solve his reflux problems. Unfortunately it hadn't, and Jack was referred to me. I quickly uncovered the difficulty. Jack was taking the Prilosec at night, on an empty stomach. This is the way we recommend taking the histamine blockers (Tagamet and Zantac) for healing stomach ulcers because they are short-acting and because a huge amount of acid is produced by the body after dinner and in the middle of the night during sleep. But Prilosec is a *long-acting* drug. And because of the way it is activated in the body, it works best when taken *with* food.

Think of it this way. For the drug to work, it needs to be switched on—like a light bulb or a television set. In my experience, the best time for this action to occur is in the morning just before breakfast. You don't have to eat a hearty meal; just a piece of bread and juice will do it. If you can't face breakfast at all, wait to take the drug just before a midmorning snack.

I gave Jack some drug samples (I don't think he would have *paid* for any medicine at this point) and asked him to come back in two weeks. "Just one pill in the morning before breakfast?" he repeated.

"One before breakfast," I said once again.

Looking doubtful, Jack left.

He was vastly improved two weeks later and had cleaned out his entire medicine cabinet. Jack has stayed on Prilosec ever since.

Terri was a high school teacher in suburban Boston. At first she was relatively healthy, only complaining about occasional incidents of mild heartburn that responded to antacids. However, at the beginning of her second pregnancy she began to experience severe fatigue and shortness of breath. Her obstetrician explained that this was not uncommon during pregnancy and that the symptoms would go away after her baby was born. Rather than improve, Terri's symptoms became much worse. In fact, six months after her delivery, her fatigue and gasping had become so severe that she was unable to return to teaching.

It was then that Terri decided to see her internist. The doctor noticed wheezing and requested tests to measure the strength of her breathing. The tests showed that her lung power was weaker than normal. Her internist diagnosed the condition as asthma and gave her medication that allowed her to breathe more normally.

At first Terri's symptoms abated, but this improvement was short-lived, and her fatigue and shortness of breath returned. She became anxious and unhappy and wondered if she was suffering from postpartum depression. As Terri put it, "I had a beautiful newborn baby and couldn't take care of him. Even the simplest tasks would make me exhausted."

Meanwhile, Terri continued taking antacids three

times a day. Like so many people we've described, she did not tell her doctor about her medication use because she didn't think taking antacids was related to a medical problem—and certainly not one that had anything to do with wheezing.

Fortunately Terri's physician, having become as frustrated as her patient, did what every good doctor should do. She didn't simply rely on what Terri told her; she probed her every action. *Something* was going on. Finally Terri mentioned her antacid use and the fact that now that she thought about it, she did have some heartburn now and then.

The internist referred her to me, and after I had given Terri a thorough examination and listened carefully to her history, I considered prescribing Prilosec. The association between heartburn and asthma was not proved, but many of Terri's symptoms were close enough to those of reflux disease to begin acid-suppressing therapy. I prescribed Prilosec, and after two weeks Terri could reduce her asthma medication in half. A month later her symptoms of wheezing and breathlessness were gone. This was the first time I, as a gastroenterologist, had ever treated an "asthma" patient although I had treated many asthmatics in the past. While I had read that asthma might be related to heartburn, I didn't have a strong enough acid-blocking medicine to test the association. The early successful results with Prilosec on breathing disorders have just begun to arouse enormous excitement in the medical community and will be discussed in the next chapter.

The Reverend Metcalf is a well-known minister in the Boston community noted for his beautifully crafted and powerfully delivered sermons. He suffered for many years with heartburn, for which he was treated on and off with Pepcid. Because of the length of time he had been affected by his disease, Reverend Metcalf was referred to me by his family doctor for a more comprehensive examination. I was asked to look at the lining of his esophagus to check for any inflammation or ulcers. The lining was normal, but Reverend Metcalf's speaking voice was not. "How long have you been hoarse?" I asked him.

"Off and on for a few months. Nothing serious."

"Nothing serious? Are you sure?"

The reverend admitted that "on occasion" he had almost lost his voice but that he had continued his Sunday services regardless. It turned out that he no longer preached without the aid of an amplifying system. Over the years the reverend had gradually increased the volume until it was almost at its maximum. "Advancing age, I guess," the reverend said, clearing his throat. It was the fourth or fifth time he'd done so since meeting me.

Normally I might have continued Reverend Metcalf on his Pepcid and increased the dose, but because of the hoarseness, I decided to prescribe Prilosec. As with asthma, we were just beginning to suspect a possible relationship between loss of voice and acid reflux, but it had not been proved. This would be an ideal opportunity for me to observe the effect of acid suppression in a patient with heartburn and hoarseness.

While I had some expectations of success, I was surprised to hear from Reverend Metcalf a week before his scheduled return visit. He told me how happy he was with his new medication. Not only was his heartburn completely gone, but several members of his congregation had said that his sermons were the best he had delivered in more than a decade. His voice was clearer and less raspy, and he was again speaking strongly without the aid of any amplification system.

On a personal level the best news of all came from my old college friend Scott. I had not seen him for a number of years, and he called unexpectedly just before the Thanksgiving holiday in 1993. He was in Boston on a business trip and wanted to take me out to dinner.

"Dinner?" I repeated.

"Dinner," he confirmed, inviting me to Legal Sea Foods, a superb local restaurant.

Scott never invited anyone to dinner. Usually he was either too sick to eat or in too much distress to enjoy his food. But he showed up promptly at the appointed time, and I barely recognized him. He had gained at least ten pounds, his face was no longer gaunt, and the familiar lines of worry and fatigue had vanished.

More surprising than Scott's appearance was his appetite. While he didn't consume as much food as, say, Diamond Jim Brady, he did manage to finish off a bowl of creamy New England clam chowder, an order of spicy fish with tomato topping, and two glasses of chardonnay. This was not the young man I remembered in college sipping milk by himself in the cafeteria—or even the adult who met me from time to time in quiet, out-of-the way locations.

Later in the dinner Scott said he was taking Prilosec.

I told him that I had worked with the drug and was happy he was responding so well. Scott then told me personal stories of which I had been unaware: of his misdiagnosis, of being referred to a psychiatrist, of spending years seeing various doctors, of even taking part in a research program comparing the results of surgery with medication.

He had started on Prilosec a year earlier and had responded within two weeks. The first sensation he noticed was an absence of pain. This is a very common occurrence. Many people with acid reflux have lived with discomfort for so long that they are surprised when their distress disappears.

As his condition improved, Scott had even ventured into a pizzeria and ordered a pie with "the works." I'm happy to say that after this initial spree he returned to a healthful low-fat diet and a good exercise program. I tell my patients who have recovered with either an H2 blocker or Prilosec that the general rules of sensible eating should still apply.

These anecdotes about patients and friends who have responded to Prilosec are intended to make a key point. The drug helps a great many people who have a wide variety of symptoms. These symptoms are part of the disease we have referred to as acid reflux, but your doctor may refer to the disorder by different names. This is due to both the complexity and the evolution of our understanding of heartburn and reflux disease. The glossary at the end of the book can help with most terminology issues. However, do not hesitate to ask your physician exactly what he or she means when you get a diagnosis. You should have a clear idea of what your condition is, how serious it is, what steps you should take to heal it, how long the condition will last, and what medication, if any, is needed. You should also know exactly how to use the medication and for what period of time it will be needed.

It may help you to write down these or any other questions and bring them with you to the doctor's office. Please do not feel embarrassed by any problem that is bothering you. Your complaint may be very important for the physician to make a correct diagnosis.

The most common questions patients ask me are: How do I know what really ails me and how can I get relief quickly and safely?

Let's answer these questions by more carefully defining how we classify your sickness. Through the years the names given to this illness and the wide array of symptoms that characterizes it have also changed, and current medical terminology is still evolving. For example, we now call the condition that the Reverend Metcalf suffered from acid laryngitis or sometimes reflux laryngitis. The term refers to the fact that the voice box is being injured by the reflux of stomach acid.

We do not have a similar descriptive term for asthma/reflux. It can be called either reflux-induced asthma or an asthmatic complication of acid reflux.

Scott's condition has now been more precisely termed. It is called erosive esophagitis and can be directly viewed by using a device called an endoscope. Erosive esophagitis is a broad term that refers to irritations of the esophagus ranging from mild to severe. In its mildest forms the disease shows up as a redness of the lining of the lower esophagus. As the severity of the ailment increases, it displays shallow ulcerations, termed erosions, hence the name erosive esophagitis. If further damage has taken place, true ulcers appear. As the damage advances, the entire surrounding of the lower esophagus looks badly scarred and inflamed.

In 1905, when this condition was first identified in the United States, we would have called this disease peptic ulcer of the esophagus. "Peptic" refers to a chemical within the stomach juices, pepsin, that helps our body digest food. But to confuse matters completely, if doctors speak today about a peptic ulcer or peptic ulcer disease, they are probably referring to *stomach* or *duodenal* ulcer.

"Peptic esophagitis" was the term used by doctors in the 1930s to describe severe heartburn. "Peptic esophagitis" or simply "esophagitis" refers to *any* acid-related irritation to the esophagus, whether it is mild or severe.

In 1950 researchers first began using the term "cardio-esophageal relaxation" to describe a state in which the sphincter "relaxes" and allows gastric juice, including acid, to surge or reflux into the esophagus. Some physicians now began referring to the disease as reflux esophagitis. The problem with the term "reflux esophagitis" is that it assumes that everyone who refluxes may develop damage to the esophagus. It was learned, however, that an enormous number of people experience reflux to some extent after eating.

Whether or not you develop esophagitis or experience heartburn symptoms depends on how much *acid* is in the refluxed material and how *long* it actually stays in contact with the esophagus. This should make perfect sense. If you have a sore on your skin, the last thing you want to do is pour an acid like lemon juice on it. If you diluted the lemon juice with plenty of water and poured it on your injury, you'd probably do little damage. But if you poured on pure lemon juice, you'd quickly feel burning. By the same token, the longer the lemon juice stayed in contact with the sore, the more severe would be your pain and the more damage to the wound.

The term "gastroesophageal reflux disease" encompasses the many factors in your illness: reflux of acid, strength of acid, duration of acid in the esophagus, and various parts of the digestive tract that are involved in the acid movement. "Gastroesophageal reflux disease," "GERD," "reflux disease," or "acid reflux" all refer to the same ailment.

Because reflux disease has surprising symptoms, is confused with other illnesses, and has constantly been misunderstood and misclassified, physicians refer to the ailment with a puzzling variety of names. Some of these names were more common in previous eras and some are a good deal easier to say than "gastroesophageal reflux disease." I've sat in on numerous discussions of acid reflux, only to hear doctors using five different terms to characterize *exactly* the same condition. More troublesome, I've sat in on numerous discussions where five completely different types of patient were characterized with the same term.

You will most likely hear your condition described as heartburn, esophagitis, acid-peptic disease, acid reflux . . . on and on with various combinations.

But the two most important points to remember are these: Serious heartburn requiring immediate treatment involves erosions or ulcers in the esophagus; uncomplicated heartburn usually will not cause erosions and is thus called nonerosive acid reflux. An internal examination is necessary to confirm the diagnosis. The presence of symptoms alone cannot establish the difference between "serious" and "uncomplicated" heartburn.

Secondly, lasting and painful heartburn may signal serious illness even if there is no evidence of erosions or ulcers. Thus you can have severe acid reflux but no esophagitis.

If you have no inflammation of the esophagus and your symptoms are not severe, the chances are good that you can be treated with Propulsid or any of the four histamine blockers—Axid, Pepcid, Tagamet, and Zantac. If you are found to have a mild inflammation, Propulsid and the H2 blockers should also be adequate.

If you have actual erosions in your esophagus or if you have tried a course of H2 blockers and still have symptoms, you most likely need Prilosec or Prevacid. I also immediately prescribe one of these drugs for patients who have been troubled for long periods of time with heartburn or when I judge the pain and discomfort of the sickness to be severe.

The treatment that's right for you can be made only in consultation with your doctor. At the end of this chapter I have included a list of questions to help you assess your ailment. By using it, you can help yourself and your physician in your search for a cure. The questions are based on my years of diagnostic experience and are meant to provide hints, not definite answers.

Why is it so important that you know and understand your illness and be aware of the proper treatment? Obviously you don't want to suffer. However, you also do not want to experience the possible complications of heartburn. In this chapter I have talked about patients who were rapidly healed by medication and went on to lead normal and productive lives. But sometimes I see people for whom I can do little. Most of them have lived many years with acid reflux and were unaware of how serious their illness could be.

Carl was forty-two years old when I saw him in the summer of 1994. He had experienced heartburn since his early teens and treated himself with antacids. He did see a physician once a year for a physical but never mentioned either his sickness or antacid use.

When he was forty-one, Carl started having difficulty breathing and was given a chest X ray, which revealed he had cancer in his lungs. Carl was referred to me to see if I could detect the source of the malignancy. Sure enough, the endoscope revealed that Carl had a cancer in his gullet associated with a condition known as Barrett's esophagus.

This very serious disease is caused by a transformation in the body known as metaplasia. In simple terms, metaplasia is the change of one kind of tissue in the body to another. The body seemingly does this in an attempt to protect itself. In the case of the esophagus, the lining of this duct alters to resemble the lining of the stomach. It undergoes this metaplasia because the body senses that the esophagus needs more protection from the irritation of stomach acid.

It is almost as if the esophagus had a built-in brain that was telling it: If you stay the way you are, you will not be able to survive, but if you turn your lining into the type found in the stomach, you will be shielded. What sounds like a protective mechanism, however, can produce disastrous complications.

The altered tissue is called Barrett's esophagus, and it is precancerous. We simply do not know yet how long it takes for this disease to form or how long it takes for cancer to develop.

Many researchers believe it takes decades of acid exposure to the lower esophagus and decades more in most patients for cancer to form. While this may be the case in the overall population, it has become evident that cancer of the lower esophagus related to Barrett's metaplasia is *the fastest-growing tumor in the United States*!

In theory the only way we could really measure how long it takes for cancer to develop would be to treat one group of patients with medication and leave the others without treatment. Needless to say, such an experiment would be highly unethical. Moreover, with the discovery of Prilosec we can heal the lining of even a badly ulcerated esophagus so that it does not *need* to transform itself into a precancerous condition.

The night after I diagnosed Carl, I had trouble sleeping and spent the hours going through studies to see if there was anything further I could do to help him. Unfortunately there was nothing; the cancer had progressed too far. The young man died about six months after I saw him, and I have asked myself many times whether earlier treatment for heartburn could have saved his life.

While I have no scientific proof, I believe it would have, and I believe there are many more people like Carl who could be helped by getting their reflux disease properly diagnosed and treated.

The best way to assess the severity of your condition is to get an endoscopy. Today an endoscopy is a relatively simple and safe procedure that takes no more than ten or fifteen minutes. A very thin, flexible tube is passed through the mouth and down through the digestive tract. At the end of this tube is a tiny light and camera that actually let us see the lining of your esophagus. (I know this does not sound pleasant, but I can assure you that with a mild anesthetic, you scarcely notice any discomfort.)

The following categories of people would be wise to discuss having this procedure with their physicians:

- Those with long histories (more than ten years) of heartburn
- Those who have heartburn that does not subside after a few weeks of therapy with either antacids or an H2 blocker
- Those with severe symptoms of heartburn

• Anyone over fifty who has a sudden onset of heartburn or other symptoms related to GERD, such as wheezing, chest pain, difficulty in swallowing, or chronic cough.

Some experts believe that endoscopy should be performed on any heartburn patient whose symptoms are severe enough to require either a high dose of an H2 blocker or Prilosec. Again we stress the importance of discussion with your doctor. My recommendation would be to go ahead with endoscopy if there is a question about the nature of your sickness.

Even if the examination does not indicate any serious problems, it may reveal an inflammation. By making sure this inflammation stays under control, you may well avoid future complications.

The H2 blocker drugs and Prilosec have proved very safe for treatment of acid reflux. The early worries that surrounded the introduction of both classes of medications were unfounded. Patients have used Tagamet and Zantac for almost two decades with no harmful effects. Prilosec has been used by patients for more than thirteen years and demonstrated a similar safety record.

Side effects are very rare. When patients were given Zantac, Prilosec, or a placebo (sugar pill), the number of reactions to each compound was the same. In other words, patients had just the same problems with medication as with no medication.

My own experience is similar. Rarely does a person complain of side effects, and I have never had to stop anyone's medication because of adverse reactions. All drugs cause changes in the chemistry of people's bodies; therefore, anyone can potentially have a bad experience with any medication, including aspirin. Older people, especially those who are taking many drugs or who have kidney, liver, or heart disease, should thoroughly discuss any medication use with their physicians or pharmacists. The elderly are more susceptible to the effects of drugs, and when many are being taken concurrently, they may interfere with one another.

Neither the H2 blockers nor Prilosec have been tested over the entire life-span of any human being. Although I can be fairly sure that no one need worry about therapy for even four or five years, no one can say what the effect of taking these medications for fifty or sixty years would be.

A cardinal rule of medicine is to assess risk versus reward. If a patient has severe acid reflux with ulcers in the esophagus (erosive esophagitis), there is no question that the benefits of continual medication or even surgery outweigh the risks of disease complications.

But as more patients with debilitating heartburn and no damage to the esophagus ask for relief, how do you assess risk versus benefit? This must be an individual choice regarding the value you place on your quality of life, your overall health, and the judgment of your doctor. Most of my patients who experience disturbing pain after stopping their medication decide to start their pills again and live a normal existence. Certainly this was the case with my friend Scott, who made it clear he would never go back to bland diets, lifestyle restrictions, and a "fire inside."

6

ASTHMA AND ACID REFLUX

The Silent Epidemic

> Asthmatics should learn to take their large daily meal at noon, in order to avoid nighttime asthma which occurs if they eat a full supper.
> —*Sir William Osler,* The Principles and Practice of Medicine, *1892*

Dorothy, a woman in her mid-thirties, had to drive more than two hours to reach the hospital where she was being treated for asthma. In need of more medical attention than her family doctor could provide, she traveled to get a new therapy being tested at a university research center eighty miles away. On an autumn day in 1993, en route to her appointment, she felt a tingling on her skin, a burning in her lungs, then a tightness in her throat. She was still thirty minutes from the hospital when her breathing became labored, with gasping and wheezing. After pulling off the highway, she grabbed her inhaler from the glove compartment and began taking in puffs of medication. Dorothy recalled the advice from her asthma education class. "Keep calm," she repeated to herself, praying that the drug would work. The wait to regain her breath seemed endless.

Dorothy is one of at least twelve million Americans who suffer from asthma. I first met her when I was involved with a study to determine whether reflux disease could be one of the triggers that set off asthmatic attacks. Although many believe that asthma is a mild condition, more than five thousand sufferers die from the illness every year. The estimated cost, including days lost from school or work, emergency room use, and hospitalizations, surpasses six billion dollars annually.

Asthma attacks can range from mild shortness of breath to frightening and uncontrollable spells of wheezing, coughing, and breathlessness. What makes the disease terrifying is that it can strike without warning and cause victims to collapse in a disoriented panic. Imagine yourself gasping for air but being unable to breathe properly. Dorothy described this feeling as "suffocating" and herself as "unable to escape an airless prison." Emergency room doctors are prepared to treat people in these situations, both with powerful medications that can open up breathing passageways and with equipment that can actually force air in and out of the lungs.

A description of the disease goes back to the Greek poet Homer, who first used the term "asthma (orthopnea)" to describe a condition of "gasping and painful breathing." Later the Greek physician Aretaeus characterized asthma by its "dry wheezing, unproductive cough and inability to sleep prone." These accurate descriptions precede our own by more than two thousand years. The Greeks also knew that asthma could be exacerbated by changes in temperature and climate and that attacks were more frequent during the fall season.

Older cultures were also familiar with the ephedra plant to treat lung problems. Emergency rooms use a drug that was developed from the same source, epinephrine, to treat asthma and allergy attacks.

The central mystery with asthma is the trigger, the substance or event that sets off an attack. Why is an asthmatic perfectly well one moment and in severe distress the next?

Western doctors in the 1700s blamed the disease, like so much else, on the rapid changes revolutionizing society: the growth of cities, crowding, speeding up of lifestyle. Symptoms of asthma and heartburn began to be linked, as made evident by a new word appearing in the English language: "hypochondriack," a person afflicted with moodiness, oversensitive skin, and poor digestion. Whatever we now think, the term "hypochondriac" was first used as a great compliment. In 1771 the *Encyclopaedia Britannica* referred to hypochondria as a "peculiar disease of the learned." In fact, this "nervous disorder" was originally reserved for those with "truly refined and exquisite temperament."

Ailments, including asthma and heartburn, were characterized by a lack of obvious physical cause; nothing was seen to be wrong with the body. So the origin of these maladies was most likely "nervous liquors"—either too much or too little "nervous tone"—or neuroses. The constriction in the airways and the food passageways causing choking, gasping, and wheezing was often described as hysteria.

Now we say that people with asthma may have underlying "emotional disorders" and that their airways are "hyperresponsive." In other words, asthmatics are more likely to become ill when in certain situations or with certain foods or substances in the air. No one currently ascribes asthma to nervous vapors, neuroses, or hysteria. The National Institutes of Health has replaced these terms with more modern ones, such as "difficult family dynamics" and "fear, anger and frustration." (Nothing's changed.) Almost at the bottom of the list of possible trigger mechanisms is evaluation of the patient for acid reflux.

For unknown reasons the "asthma population" has recently increased, in terms of both hospitalizations and numbers of deaths. According to Dr. Michael Kaliner of the National Institutes of Health, "In terms of human suffering, asthma is right at the top of the list. U.S. cases have probably gone up by 100 percent in the last two decades and the death rate has almost doubled in the last ten years."

Many questions and controversies exist about what has caused this increase and about the disease itself. We have long known about many asthmatic triggers: allergies, poor air quality, and viral and bacterial infections. In addition, the disease is associated with pregnancy, an overactive thyroid, inflamed sinuses, changes in climate and altitude, and even depression.

When these triggers are present, the airways are more likely to become inflamed. The inflammation causes swelling and narrowing of the respiratory passages, often accompanied by the production of mucus and fluid that further obstruct the ability to breathe. This obstruction is responsible for such symptoms as wheezing and coughing—signs that the body is struggling to pull in and, to a greater extent, let out more air. Inflammation also causes muscles in the breathing passages to contract violently—tightening and untightening—causing asthmatics to feel that a noose is being tightened around their necks. Usually these symptoms can be controlled, but on occasion, even with medication, the asthmatic attack continues, making emergency treatment essential.

The respiratory system of an asthmatic is more easily irritated than that of a person who does not suffer from the disease. Cigarette smoke, whether inhaled directly or secondhand, may cause an asthmatic to have problems breathing, as can cold air and exercise.

Patients are usually treated with medications that reduce tissue inflammation, such as steroid inhalers (Aerobid, Beclovent, and Vanceril), oral steroids (prednisone), or cromolyn sodium (Intal). Other medications that relax the airway muscles are called bronchodilators (Ventolin, Proventil, Maxair) and theophylline (Theo-Dur).

According to the National Institutes of Health, patients with mild and occasional attacks should be started on an "inhaled" bronchodilator. If attacks become more severe, an inhaled anti-inflammatory drug should also be used. (An inhaled drug is a spray or powder that goes directly to the irritated passageways. A "systemic" drug generally is a pill that is swallowed. Doctors often prefer inhaled drugs because they cause fewer side effects.)

Many asthma patients are not easy to categorize, and if the severity of their disease changes, they may need different amounts and types of medication throughout their lives. But since inflammation is the underlying cause of the illness, everyone agrees that the best way of treating asthma is to *eliminate the irritating trigger*.

What has been discovered and now clearly proved is that the reflux of stomach acid, sometimes accompanied by heartburn, is one of the sources of inflammation that set off asthmatic attacks. Dorothy found this out quickly at the medical center where she was being treated. She kept a diary of everything she ate and noted

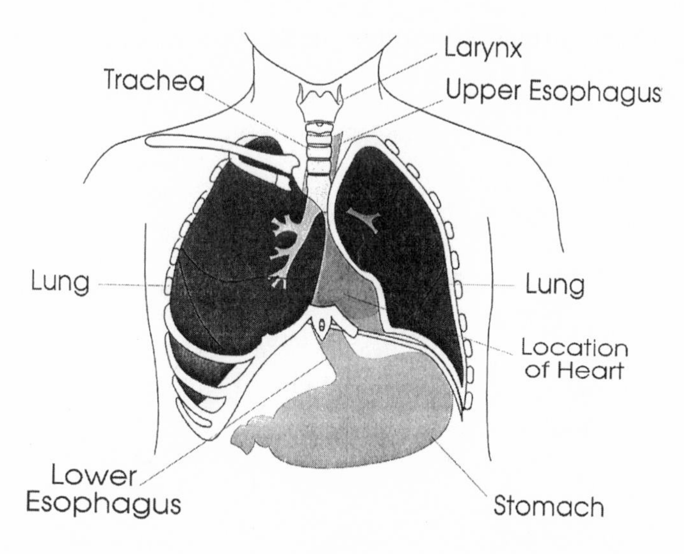

fig 2

the times of her wheezing and shortness of breath. She found that her asthma attacks coincided with both heartburn symptoms and the reflux of gastric juice into her esophagus.

It should not be difficult to imagine why this happens when you look at figure 2. As you can see, the esophagus, stomach, and lungs are adjacent to one another. As I have already explained, the esophagus is not equipped to handle acid and can be easily damaged by it. The same is true of the lungs and air passageways, especially among asthmatics, who are even *more* sensitive to irritants.

We call asthma-related reflux disease the silent epidemic because it is very serious, very prevalent, potentially life-threatening, and not widely known. There are many reasons for its obscurity. Asthma-related reflux is difficult to diagnose and until recently has been nearly impossible to treat without surgery. In some ways it is just as mysterious and invisible today as asthma was in the seventeenth century. Indeed, it is ignored.

In April 1993 the American Medical Association held a major press conference to educate journalists and the public about the increasing problem of asthma. The experts correctly pointed out that millions of Americans with the disease remain undiagnosed. They also indicated important features in asthma management: "drug treatment, environmental control measures (particularly tobacco smoke) and patient education."

However, the possibility that acid reflux could contribute to asthma was not mentioned. In October 1994 the *Annals of Internal Medicine,* the official publication of the American College of Physicians (a prestigious journal that defines medical diagnosis in America), made no mention at all of acid reflux as a potential trigger of asthma.

You might conclude that people like Dorothy, in whom the association between reflux disease and asthma has been proved, are few or that research has not been carried out. You would be wrong on both counts. Carefully designed studies indicate that between 34 and 89 percent of asthmatics have acid reflux. These same studies show that *half* of all asthmatics could be either significantly improved or actually cured with antireflux therapy.

Thus the number of people who would benefit in the United States alone is more than six million. And research to demonstrate this has been going on for years at major medical centers. In fact, the first modern scientist to suspect the link between lung problems and digestion was Sir William Osler, regarded as the father of present-day medicine and one of the principals of Johns Hopkins University. Osler noted that symptoms of indigestion were related to an increase in asthmatic attacks. As early as 1887 European doctors also noted that repeated episodes of pneumonia and other severe lung diseases were related to the swelling and inflammation of the esophagus.

No one followed up on these observations, probably because it was impossible to examine the upper digestive tract with detail or measure accurately the movement or effect of stomach acid. In the late 1950s and 1960s, however, diagnostic tools that could accurately detect acid in the esophagus were invented. Soon thereafter physicians reported that acid reflux correlated with lung disease.

A chest specialist named John I. Kennedy noted in 1960 that patients entering the Frenchay Hospital in Bristol, England, had both crippling breathing problems and reflux disease. He found that when some lung patients were surgically treated for their reflux, the pulmonary symptoms disappeared. He also made another significant observation: Among patients with acid reflux and lung disease, only 40 percent had heartburn. For this reason he cautioned doctors about silent reflux, by which he meant reflux not accompanied by heartburn or related digestive symptoms.

Throughout the 1960s other surgeons confirmed Kennedy's findings. Many observed that if a patient suffered from acid reflux and lung problems, and no obvious cause could be found for the breathing distress (such as an allergy), the problem could be solved by treating the acid reflux. It was also established that if patients with both conditions *improved* after acid reflux treatment, reflux caused the asthma.

The problem was that no simple way existed to test or treat patients. Only sufferers with severe lung or reflux disease came to the attention of surgeons, and the number who underwent operations was relatively small. Most asthma and reflux patients do not have disease severe enough to require surgery, nor could the health care system of any country handle the quantity of relatively difficult operations that would be necessary.

Because Kennedy and other investigators were chest specialists, they dealt mostly with patients who had severe breathing problems. However, in 1976 Dr. Edward Mays, writing in the *Journal of the American Medical Association,* noted that a large number of people with a wide variety of breathing problems such as asthma might also have a disorder caused by acid reflux. Mays looked at patients with asthma and reflux, many of whom had been treated with respiratory medication. Like all asthma researchers, he was trying to find what triggered an asthmatic attack.

Because his patients' symptoms were not severe enough to require surgery, they were given the most potent drug treatment of that time for acid reflux. The results were not conclusive, although Mays did see some improvement in his patients' asthma symptoms. He recommended an intensive trial of antireflux therapy for asthmatics in whom no other triggering factors could be found. He also cautioned physicians to watch for silent reflux disease, which like Dr. Kennedy, he defined as reflux without the classic symptom of heartburn.

Despite the warning, two problems remained. Physicians did not have any medication powerful enough to halt acid production sufficiently to have an effect on reflux-induced asthma. Secondly, they did not have an easily available instrument with which to make the diagnosis.

The first problem looked as if it might be solved with the release of Tagamet and Zantac. When these drugs were initially tested on asthmatics, the patients improved, but not enough to encourage widespread use.

In the early 1990s more studies were done with higher doses of Zantac and Tagamet to see if such regimens would work on patients who had severe acid reflux with breathing problems. The results of these experiments were compared with surgery, and it was found that surgical treatment of acid reflux associated with asthma was superior to drug treatment. With antireflux surgery, 75 percent were cured but even with a high dose of Zantac a disappointing number of asthmatics (10 percent) were improved.

Why had surgery proved so effective with the asthmatic complications of reflux disease while drugs had been largely ineffective? The most plausible explanation is the extreme sensitivity of the affected organs to stomach acid. As I explained, even high doses of Zantac and Tagamet are only partially effective in healing an inflamed esophagus and are even less effective in healing more extensive esophageal ulcers.

This is because the lining of the esophagus has been so damaged that if even a trace of stomach acid touches it, the sore continues. The situation is similar in the air passageways of asthmatics. Minuscule acid exposure can trigger an asthmatic attack or make the inflammation worse. What is needed is therapy that prevents *any* stomach acid from getting to these extremely sensitive parts of the body. This is what happens with successful antireflux operations and why surgeons get good response rates. Until the development of Prilosec, no drug could duplicate this response. With this medication, a potent medicine was available that worked *continually, night and day*.

Nonetheless, the problem of how to diagnose the patient with reflux-induced asthma remained. As both

Kennedy and Mays pointed out, the reflux is not accompanied by the obvious symptom of heartburn. Nor does reflux-induced asthma often cause damage to the esophagus. Therefore, physicians cannot see it by using an endoscope. Detecting this silent disease can now be done only two ways: by using the relatively new and sophisticated diagnostic instrument called a pH probe or by actually shutting off the acid with medication and observing the result.

The pH probe was developed in the latter part of the 1960s to detect the presence and potency of acid in the esophagus. The term "pH" refers to the potency measurement. The probe is more accurate than the endoscope for diagnosing acid reflux because it actually measures the acid concentration in the esophagus. The device consists of a tiny tube that is placed down the throat and into the gullet. At the end of the tube is an electronic sensor that measures the presence and strength (pH) of acid. The signals from the sensor are transmitted to a box with a recorder that a patient wears for about twenty-four hours. After this period the device is removed and the results are analyzed by a computer. Unlike an endoscope, which allows the doctor to see the esophagus, the pH probe is an electronic tool in which no actual viewing of the body is done. Its function is to measure acid content and potency, not to view tissue.

If a patient has acid reflux but shows no damage to the esophagus and has no symptoms of heartburn (silent reflux), the pH probe may still detect and measure acid. A computer terminal displays how much acid was present in the esophagus and how potent it was. The pH probe is particularly helpful to assess patients with atypical symptoms of acid reflux, such as asthma, chest pain, and hoarseness, because many do not have symptoms of heartburn or esophagitis.

This was the case with Dorothy, the woman mentioned at the beginning of this chapter. Tests at the university center easily confirmed she had difficulty breathing. They also confirmed that she had no inflammation or ulcers in her esophagus. She was asked detailed questions about her personal and medical history: medications she had taken, illnesses, deaths in the family, living and working conditions, exercise, emotional relationships, and stress.

Her asthma had developed when she was twenty-two for no apparent reason. At first it was mild and easily treatable with a Ventolin inhaler, but through the years it had steadily gotten worse, requiring two hospitalizations and four trips to the emergency room. The asthma appeared regardless of seasons, living conditions, medications, or any other factors the doctors could ascertain.

By the age of thirty-six Dorothy was in a desperate situation. She was using powerful antiasthma drugs and the side effects were showing. The prednisone tablets had caused her weight to increase twenty pounds, made her nervous, and swollen her face. Her husband pointed out an advertisement in the local newspaper asking for volunteers to study a new asthma therapy. Making the trip was Dorothy's biggest worry. She hated to drive long distances for fear of being too far away from her family physician and her clinic's emergency room.

Although Dorothy had a very supportive family, she was asked about "marital problems" every time she appeared for emergency treatment. A number of times since she had developed asthma as an adult, health care professionals had prescribed antianxiety medications, such as Valium and Xanax.

Dorothy used them on occasion, but they never helped her illness. Actually she and her husband got along well, both her children were honors students, and she led an active and productive life at home and work, where she tutored for her church.

After giving this detailed personal history, Dorothy received a lung function test to measure her breathing and an endoscopy. The pH probe was then administered, and during the twenty-four hours of the test Dorothy was asked to keep a diary of everything she ate as well as a record of her emotional state and breathing problems. After the results of the test were analyzed, it was clear that Dorothy had very high levels of acid in her esophagus and that every time the acid level became higher, symptoms of asthma became worse.

She was treated with Prilosec twice a day to eliminate all stomach acid from coming in contact with either her airways or esophagus. By the eighth week of therapy Dorothy had cut her inhaler use in half, and by the end of the three-month medication course she needed only occasional asthma medication. Obviously acid reflux was triggering many of Dorothy's breathing problems.

Careful experiments with patients such as Dorothy show that asthmatic patients have malfunctioning valves between the stomach and esophagus that more easily allows acid reflux. These people also have problems with digestion. A careful review of all the research that has looked at the relationship between acid reflux and asthma indicate that *half* of all asthmatics have GERD as the principal trigger.

If you think you may be one of them, the best way to start the diagnosis is simple. First, consider whether you have heartburn. I often find that because patients are so frightened of their asthma, they overlook something as common as heartburn. Secondly, talk to your doctor and relate all your symptoms as precisely and completely as possible.

Does your asthma get worse after consuming meals? Do certain foods make your asthma worse? Is it particularly bad at night? Is it affected by your body position? If you have heartburn, how severe is it? How often does it occur? Does it coincide with breathing problems?

Do you know what is triggering your asthma? Many asthmatics know the cause of their illness—for example, allergies. But many asthmatics do not know what triggers their disease. These are the people who would do well to explore acid reflux as a possible cause of their asthmatic attacks.

Other groups of people who should look at this possibility are patients who have not had success being treated with usual asthma medication, patients in whom the disease has been severe, and patients who have had the disease for many years.

Your doctor may first suggest an X-ray test. In this test the patient swallows barium (a liquid coating) and is then given an X ray of the lower and upper esophagus. This test helps a physician determine whether acid materials may be contributing to asthma. However, if nothing shows on the X ray, you may still have acid reflux. Even so, I recommend this test as a starting point because it is painless, easy to perform, and relatively inexpensive.

Endoscopy, an important tool in the evaluation of heartburn, is less valuable in the diagnosis of reflux-induced asthma. It is common to have symptoms of asthma without any irritation to the esophagus (esophagitis). This fact is one of many that contributes to the confusion about reflux-induced asthma. Most doctors assume that if a patient has no physical esophageal damage, serious reflux disease is not present. But in the case of asthma acid reflux can be *life-threatening* and still show nothing with the endoscope.

As I've said, the most definitive test to measure the complications of asthma and GERD is the twenty-four-hour pH probe. But the probe is complicated, expensive, somewhat uncomfortable, and not widely available. It is more likely to remain primarily a research tool than a practical diagnostic device.

What I now advocate more often is empirical testing: using a drug at high dosages to see if it works on a disease. This approach has the advantage of not only diagnosing patients but treating their problems at the same time. The most recent studies with asthmatic patients point to using a high dose of Prilosec—one capsule two times a day—for two to three months. The best time to take the pills is before breakfast and before dinner to ensure the maximum effect of the drug. This might not be the dose used to treat the disease, but to make a diagnosis, acid needs to be shut off almost completely.

Some of the best current research on this condition is being been carried out by Dr. Susan Harding, a lung specialist from the University of Alabama; Dr. Joel Richter, a digestive disease specialist from the Cleveland Clinic; and Dr. Stephen Sontag, of the Hines, Illinois, Veterans Administration Hospital. In a study presented in May 1994 Harding and Richter found that Prilosec improved the health of 73 percent of patients who had acid reflux and asthma.

They emphasized that for the medication to be effective, stomach acid had to be halted far longer than in ordinary heartburn patients. Relief of symptoms was found to take as long as three months. During this period patients should continue to use their conventional asthma medication. If antireflux therapy works, asthmatics will probably first notice less need for their usual pills or inhalers.

Research now indicates that after a two- or three-month period of Prilosec treatment, many asthmatics with reflux disease can decrease or even eliminate conventional medication. Anyone with lung illness who undertakes this therapy should do so only under the close supervision of a physician.

One of the most common triggers of asthma is exercise. Many people are afraid that activity will cause an asthmatic attack and avoid either sports or any exertion linked with wheezing and breathing difficulty. However, many cases of "exercise-induced" asthma can be easily cured and controlled by using acid-suppressing medication.

Exercise causes increased acid reflux because it slows the digestion of food and often makes it easier for stomach acid to reach the esophagus. The acidic mixture of food and acid triggers an inflammation in the airways that leads to the typical symptom of reflux, heartburn, and to the atypical symptoms of wheezing and shortness of breath. Many people don't notice the heartburn because they are far more concerned about regaining normal breathing.

The unfortunate result is that those who exercise, whether they are occasional tennis players or Olympic athletes, are not properly diagnosed and treated for acid reflux. Instead most rely solely on conventional asthma medications. This is particularly troubling among athletes who must comply with various rules prohibiting the use of certain drugs. The International Olympic Committee bans bronchodilator pills (Proventil and

Ventolin) and some inhaled asthma medication.

Recreational athletes, while not banned from using these drugs, find it distressing to have to carry inhalers with them when they work out. Many find that breathing problems either worsen their performance or force them to curtail their activity severely.

I have helped a number of these people, one of whom is a young runner named Chris. He came to see me because he had developed difficulty swallowing, as well as wheezing and shortness of breath. I learned that Chris had recently altered his running schedule from morning to evening and that this change had brought on his symptoms. An endoscopic examination confirmed what I suspected. Chris had an inflammation of the esophagus caused in part by the fact that during the day he often had large, late business lunches. The partially digested food mixed with stomach acid that surged upward when he ran.

I immediately prescribed Prilosec for three months to heal the inflammation. Chris quickly got relief from his symptoms and regained his previous level of performance. To prevent recurrence of his problem, I have asked Chris either to run in the mornings or to take antireflux medication (Tagamet) one hour before running.

We do not know how many people with exercise-induced asthma actually suffer from acid reflux. We do know two things: Exercise is a frequent cause of breathing problems and a frequent cause of heartburn. Heartburn patients are much more likely than the normal population to experience wheezing and shortness of breath during exercise. Therefore, anyone who engages in physical activity and suffers from continual heartburn should seek treatment for his or her acid reflux.

Recall, however, that heartburn may not be present among those with acid reflux and breathing problems.

These people can either go through more extensive testing or try antireflux medication to see if their wheezing and shortness of breath improve.

To summarize, asthma is a frequent complication of acid reflux from which many suffer but for which few are treated. Asthmatics should consider further medical attention if they have any of the following difficulties:

- Symptoms of acid reflux: heartburn, chest or abdominal pain, bloating, pain, or difficulty swallowing
- Wheezing, coughing, shortness of breath that occur after meals or in association with heartburn
- Continuing asthma despite therapy with conventional breathing medication (steroids, bronchodilators, theophylline)

Asthmatics who know what triggers their attacks, like allergens, pollutants, and seasonal changes, will probably not have acid reflux as a primary irritant. Nonetheless, even in this population patients with heartburn should pay extra attention to keeping their reflux disease under control. On the other hand, patients who have had continual asthma problems with no identifiable trigger may wish to consider evaluation for acid reflux—especially if there has been poor response to conventional breathing medication.

Identifying and controlling asthma are a major public health problem, and I believe that acid reflux–induced asthma is a large component of this epidemic. Treatment for this condition is now relatively simple and the results potentially life-altering, if not lifesaving.

7

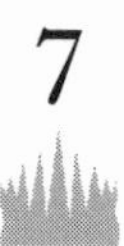

ACID REFLUX

Ear, Nose, and Throat Complications

> Red wine . . . bindeth the belly and maketh hoarsenesse.
>
> —*Thomas Cogan,* The Haven of Health, *1598*

> Figs are useful in Hoarseness and Coughs
>
> —*John Arbuthnot,* Rules of Diet, *1732*

Joseph was a successful trial lawyer in Los Angeles, well known for his spellbinding jury summations. He seldom lost a case and was consulted by defendants throughout the United States. In 1988, without any warning, he began feeling a slight pain when he spoke. Joseph tried rest and relaxation, gargling with salt water, herbal teas, even chicken soup, but his voice continued to deteriorate. He went to numerous doctors and was given medications such as antihistamines to dry up the mucus in his throat, antibiotics for infection, and prednisone for swelling—but nothing worked.

Joseph was eventually forced to take a leave of absence from his law firm and decline all further work. He was hoarse much of the time and lost his voice completely for days. Joseph lapsed into depression as he considered his bleak existence and future life: an inability to continue working; loss of his law practice, self-esteem, and income. Even if he changed professions, what could he do without being able to speak?

We do not know how many people are affected by severe hoarseness and loss of voice, but the numbers are likely in the millions. For many people like Joseph whose voices are directly related to their jobs, the problem is incapacitating. Teachers, lawyers, clergymen, singers, executives, receptionists—the list goes on at length—all rely on their voices.

As with asthma, many people do not consider a voice problem serious, but not only can it threaten a livelihood, but it may lead to ulcers around the voice box and either precancerous or cancerous developments. These potential or actual malignancies are not the result of an occasional sore throat or laryngitis but a problem that occurs because of a condition that has existed on a regular basis for years.

Unlike swelling of the esophagus (esophagitis), swelling around the vocal cords (laryngitis) is relatively easy to diagnose. Sometimes the condition comes on gradually, the voice losing power over a few days until it is barely a whisper. In other instances, the voice becomes low and gravelly, especially in the morning. You wake up, try to speak, and a faint rumbling comes out. "People call me sir, on the phone," one female patient told me. "My mother thinks I growl like a dog."

The severity of the condition is partly subjective and may depend on how critical a normal voice is to you. For a person like Joseph, even slight hoarseness was so serious he could not practice his profession. I have had patients who were singers, actors, and announcers who came for treatment, despite sounding almost normal, because they feared that even the mildest cases of laryngitis would ruin their careers.

Other patients live a regular life with a constant mild voice problem. Some even think it's sexy. The so-called Bogart-Bacall syndrome is named after Humphrey Bogart and Lauren Bacall, both of whom had low, husky voices that gave shivers to movie audiences in the 1940s. Note that the two performers were often photographed through an alluring haze of cigarette smoke and that Bogart later died of lung cancer.

Many causes of laryngitis have long been known: voice abuse (yelling and shouting), infections caused by viruses and bacteria, allergies, and continual inhalation of irritating substances, such as industrial fumes or cigarette smoke. Loss of voice heals with voice rest, treatment of the infection, avoidance of allergens, and keeping away from throat irritants, such as smoke and alcohol.

But a different form of hoarseness is chronic and will not respond to these treatments. The medical name for this condition is reflux laryngitis or acid laryngitis, and it is caused by stomach acid moving into the voice box, or larynx. It is a frequent occurrence and often seen by ear, nose, and throat (ENT) doctors.

Reflux-related diseases of the ear, nose, and throat are closely linked to lung diseases, and both sets of maladies share many symptoms. The reason is that before acid can move into the lungs, it must pass through a gateway known as the larynx. The larynx houses the delicate tissues known as vocal cords that allow us to create speech. When the lining of the larynx or the cords themselves are irritated, speaking becomes difficult or impossible.

The relationship between acid reflux and hoarseness has been as difficult to establish as the link between acid reflux and asthma, and for similar reasons. The voice box is in a well-protected part of the upper airway and until recently has been difficult to examine closely. Only since the 1960s has diagnostic equipment existed that could closely and directly view this organ, and only during the last few years have we had devices that could measure acid in this region of the body.

The first problem with seeing the larynx is that you need a source of illumination small enough to pass to the end of the throat. Imagine this passageway as a long dark tunnel lined with sensitive tissues. The initial crude attempts to look into this shaft were made in the middle 1800s with candlelight or a burning mixture of alcohol and turpentine. Such devices no doubt did little to encourage those with voice disorders to see a doctor. The second problem is getting the light source down the patients' throats and not burn or choke them to death.

An early researcher named Kussmaul created a long tube by studying the techniques and equipment of sword swallowers. No record exists that he ever used his device in medical practice.

Thomas Edison's invention of the electric light bulb at least partially solved the illumination problem, and as early as 1902 doctors had managed to connect an incandescent lamp to a pipe flexible enough to get down the throat. A year later a noted expert, Dr. L. A. Coffin, aroused enormous excitement among his colleagues when he presented a paper linking problems of the "upper air passages" with those in the digestive tract.

Coffin stated that he was "struck by the large number of patients" with voice problems in his practice who complained of postnasal drip. He believed the cause to be related to the contents of the stomach.

Coffin correctly pointed out that this condition was overlooked because his patients "gave no symptoms pointing to gastric disorder." This is the same complaint of silent reflux about which lung physicians wrote. A Dr. J. A. Thompson is on record as stating that he had noted many cases of hoarseness "which had proved absolutely rebellious to treatment until too much acid in the stomach had been diagnosed and properly treated." Dr. Thompson further pointed out that reflux during sleep was also responsible for sore throat and runny nose.

Like Osler's observation about food and acid, these early guesses could be neither proved nor disproved. Coffin had no means of carefully examining the larynx, and his remedy for acid disorders left a great deal to be desired: calomel, chlorate of potash, mercury, chalk, colonic irrigations, and bicarbonate of soda. The theory behind this therapy was both to administer antacids and to "purge" the patient—"clean out internal poisons." But by so doing, doctors were giving their patients toxic substances.

In 1968 Drs. J. Cherry and S. I. Margulies first scientifically demonstrated the relationship between ulcerations of the voice box and severe reflux disease. Interestingly, although the patients they saw had hoarseness or loss of voice, none had heartburn. They were treated with diet changes, elevation of the heads of their beds, and large doses of antacids—and each patient showed some improvement. Laboratory experiments a short time after proved that the vocal cords in animals could be badly damaged by the effects of stomach acid.

A few years later researchers demonstrated a link among reflux disease, severe laryngitis, and a condition called globus sensation. Globus sensation is a feeling of a lump in the back of the throat. This association was surprising to many physicians because it showed that stomach acid could travel far higher up through the body than anyone had previously thought possible.

In my own practice I sometimes see patients with *dental problems*. The stomach acid has traveled up through the throat into the back of the mouth. This in turn causes erosions of the back of the teeth.

While antacids were the mainstay of treatment for acid laryngitis and demonstrated some success in the 1960s, they were not strong enough to allow the vocal cords to heal completely. Even small amounts of gastric juice can inflame the voice box, and therefore, far greater total acid suppression is needed if reflux-related hoarseness is to be treated. This is exactly the case with asthma. It takes only a small amount of acid to trigger an attack, and antacids do not have the power to neutralize acid sufficiently.

In the 1970s and 1980s doctors prescribed Tagamet and Zantac to treat reflux laryngitis. The results were only partially successful because like antacids, the H2 blocker medications could not suppress acid long and potently enough to allow vocal cord healing. In the early 1990s physicians began to experiment with Prilosec, which, for many patients like the trial lawyer Joseph, represented a last chance.

Joseph sought treatment for his condition at a large

medical center in Boston. It was now two years since he had entered a courtroom, and he had all but given up the practice of law. Joseph was diagnosed by a new electronic device that was capable of measuring acid concentration, or pH, in the area around the base of the throat. Another instrument that uses a miniature camera actually allowed specialists to see and photograph the swelling around Joseph's vocal cords. When the results of both tests were combined, they conclusively showed that the laryngitis was caused by acid reflux.

Joseph's personal history did not indicate an obvious disease origin. His lifestyle, for example, was the portrait of moderation. He did not smoke, drank an occasional beer, and lived on "California cuisine," consisting of salads, vegetables, and baked skinless chicken breasts. (He admitted to a Japanese mushroom pizza with goat cheese once a week and was assured this was unlikely to have caused a total loss of voice.) As for his weight, Joseph was fashionably Southern California thin. He had never experienced heartburn.

Joseph was told to take two pills a day of Prilosec, one in the morning and one in the evening before meals. The goal was to eliminate almost all stomach acid production. Joseph went back to Los Angeles carrying several boxes of the new drug and hoped it would work. He was told that it might take as much as six months for his damaged vocal cords to heal.

Acid laryngitis is still not well understood. As with asthma-related reflux, a patient can have an enormous amount of stomach acid pumping up through the digestive and respiratory system and have no irritation to the esophagus. No one is sure how the damaging acidic mixture gets into the lungs or the voice box without harming the esophagus, but there is no doubt that it does.

Moreover, we are not sure why many patients with reflux disease and asthma or hoarseness do not have heartburn. However, there is an intriguing difference in the experience of symptoms. Heartburn patients almost always feel worse when they lie down. But laryngitis patients generally feel worse when they are *standing up*.

One of the problems faced by patients with any form of reflux disease is knowing which medical specialist to see. If you have a combination of hoarseness, coughing, wheezing, heartburn, and asthma (as many patients do), you might be referred to, or decide to see, an ENT specialist or a gastroenterologist, like me. Chances are you will go to the doctor who is expert in treating the symptom that is giving you the most trouble. For example, a patient with severe heartburn but only occasional hoarseness is likely to see me, a gastroenterologist. Such a patient might mention his hoarseness only if I specifically asked about it. He might not think of it as a medical problem. On the other hand, patients with bad asthma (but mild heartburn) almost always see lung specialists first. And patients whose chief complaint is related to acid laryngitis go to ENT experts. Each of these specialists may or may not be aware of *all* the consequences of acid reflux. The specialist is trained to be alert for a particular set of symptoms. Few ENT physicians will probe as deeply into stomach problems as will a digestive disease specialist. (Nor do I, as a gastroenterologist, ask as many detailed questions about the vocal cords.)

My point is that the symptoms of people with various forms of reflux disease may not differ as much as we think. If a physician asks, "Are you absolutely sure you've never experienced heartburn? Are you sure your voice is all right?" the emphasis in the question may determine the patient's answer. I had a very wise professor who explained to me that if a doctor looks hard enough, he or she will find a problem even if it's not there.

Like witnesses on the courtroom stand, patients answer leading questions with statements like "Come to think of it, I did have trouble with my . . ." (Fill in the difficulty.) So patients who have lung problems talk about breathing problems to the lung specialist, patients who have stomach problems talk about heartburn problems to the gastroenterologist, and patients with laryngitis talk about voice problems to the throat specialist. It is entirely possible that each patient has a very similar group of symptoms characteristic of reflux disease that he or she is either not aware of or not encouraged to speak about.

A number of things are at work. Patients focus on the problem that most bothers them; specialists who deal with that problem tend to focus their attention on treating that particular problem. Further complicating matters and making diagnosis difficult are the fact that one person can have two illnesses whose symptoms overlap. Someone can have asthmatic wheezing triggered by allergens *and* by reflux disease. Loss of voice can result from voice abuse and acid reflux. Many times one ailment will make another ailment worse. Among asthmatics, coughing and wheezing exacerbate reflux. Acid reflux may also worsen asthma. Thus the lung specialist who diagnoses asthma is correct, as is the gastroenterologist who diagnoses reflux.

It is not uncommon for patients with acid reflux to be

trapped in a vicious cycle. That is what happened to a political leader I know who was running for state office. He was giving speeches twenty hours a day, eating rich foods at all hours, and not getting proper rest. After a month of this routine he became hoarse. He had indeed overworked his vocal cords. But the weakened cords were now more susceptible to the injurious effects of refluxed acid. The result was eventual loss of voice. Three days before an important television debate the politician came to see a group of specialists. (A true political leader, he did not like to do anything without at least three people conferring and agreeing.)

The politician was told to rest his voice completely and was prescribed Prilosec twice a day. He recovered by the time of the debate and did an excellent job against his opponent. The speed with which Prilosec worked in this instance was unusual. Generally it takes months for those with severe laryngitis to heal, as was the case with the trial lawyer Joseph. For him the healing process was excruciatingly slow. Indeed, Joseph's wife was the first to notice. Her husband's voice slowly lost its raspy tone and became fuller and louder. The improvement was most obvious in the morning. Before medical treatment Joseph (in his wife's words) woke up "sounding like a frog" on his good days and "sounding like a broken foghorn" on his bad ones. After one month he began to talk with normal volume, and after three months he could speak with the resonance and emotion that had characterized his trial summations.

Joseph returned to work in six months and successfully resumed his career. He no longer takes Prilosec but has been maintained on Zantac. When he feels his voice weakening, Joseph immediately resumes Prilosec until he is healed.

The general advice we give people with hoarseness and loss of voice is similar to that given to those with asthma. The first step is lifestyle modification. The most serious voice irritant is smoking, and even exposure to secondhand smoke can worsen the condition. When smoking is combined with alcohol, the voice box is further affected. The simultaneous use of tobacco and alcohol is worse than each used separately.

It is unlikely that people with laryngitis will do well with simple antacids, although these drugs may be useful in mild cases. More powerful acid-suppressing therapy should be considered by those:

- Who have laryngitis unrelated to any infection or other obvious medical cause (such as allergy)
- Who have hoarseness and loss of voice that are affecting their daily functioning
- Who have had laryngitis for a long period of time or who have had the disease on and off over long periods

Another clue to acid laryngitis is difficulty in swallowing. This problem occurs in about one third of patients with reflux disease and can be caused by the irritation and swelling of the esophagus or throat from exposure to gastric juices. Heartburn may or may not be present. If it is, that is an important clue to the cause of hoarseness, especially if it is accompanied by constant clearing of the throat and a chronic cough. As I emphasized before, *please* tell your doctor about your heartburn—as well as your throat problems—even if the heartburn seems only a minor nuisance to you.

It is important to underscore the individual nature of classifying the severity and recommending treatment for voice problems. Trial lawyers, singers, or political leaders may be far more concerned about laryngitis than those who do not use their voices professionally, and they may want more powerful therapy. On the other hand, many people can more easily tolerate hoarseness—for example, a young athlete who was referred to me with mild heartburn and a "husky" voice. A short course of antacids cured him fully. What is interesting is that he was actually sorry that his voice had returned to normal. He told me that the husky voice went along with his masculine image and helped his social life.

In medicine, as in everything else, you can't please everyone.

Voice complications, like asthmatic difficulties, have always been thought to be linked to the emotions. We all have seen movies in which people are so frightened they cannot speak, and the classic form of nervousness is the "lump in the throat." It can precede any stressful event and has been used by comedians to get laughs since the ancient Greek dramatist Aristophanes wrote his comedy *The Frogs*. (Ichabod Crane, one of the first American literary heroes, was described as always having such a lump.)

Physicians originally thought the condition affected women because they believed that the uterus was a free-floating ball that would move up into the throat during emotional periods. There was actually a medical term, *Globus hystericus,* deriving from the Latin word *globus* ("ball") and the Greek word for "uterus," *hystera*.

Like the "hypochondriack," the "hysteric" often had a series of symptoms linked to nervous causes, and in the nineteenth century a large body of medicine grew up around treating patients—especially women—with these symptoms. From the backboards of horse-drawn wagons, doctors peddled elixirs that bore colorful names like Dr. Girard's Ginger Brandy and promised to cure nearly every imaginable ill.

These potions had a few things in common: some form of narcotic, such as opium, and a good jolt of alcohol. (Codeine is still the most effective remedy for cough, though you now need a prescription to obtain it, and alcohol is still found in many over-the-counter cold remedies.) Thus, like most historical remedies, they accomplished the twin goals of calming you down and making you feel better—at least temporarily.

Modern scientists have researched lump in the throat and concluded that it is rarely an emotional syndrome. The most common symptoms accompanying the globus sensation are hoarseness and heartburn. The most recent studies indicate that a majority of patients may respond to therapy for reflux disease with drugs that block acid production, like Tagament and Prilosec, or digestion-aiding drugs, such as Propulsid.

Another throat and nose condition related to acid reflux is postnasal drip. This malady is commonly caused by infection and allergies, and patients are frequently treated with antihistamines, steroids, and antibiotics. None of these treatments will work if the underlying cause is reflux.

Steve was a young patient of mine who was an optometrist. I initially treated him for a mild duodenal ulcer that healed quickly. But Steve was bothered by other, more vague stomach problems, for which I could find no cause.

One day Steve announced that his fiancée had threatened to call off their wedding if his medical problem continued. I thought Steve was referring to his stomach problem, but he then told me he had terrible postnasal drip and throat clearing that drove his fiancée "crazy." I prescribed the usual treatments of antihistamines (Seldane and later Claritin), as well as steroid nasal sprays, but neither form of therapy worked.

Because stomach pain remained a complaint, and I knew about throat complications of acid reflux, I tried Prilosec. Within a few weeks the throat clearing and postnasal drip had ceased. Interestingly so had Steve's snoring. I do not know of any research about snoring and reflux disease, and it is very difficult to find out which of my patients snore because they are unaware of what they sound like when asleep. But I have heard on occasion from a few spouses who report that snoring disappears when reflux-related asthma and throat problems are treated. As a physician I don't like to recommend a treatment that has not been scientifically tested, but if the noise level in your bedroom is a problem, you have little to lose with a course of antireflux therapy.

This same therapy may also work on severe hiccups, a disorder that sounds as if it were invented by the Marx Brothers but is very real, potentially dangerous, and fortunately rare. Acid reflux has been associated with hiccups, but as in the case of asthma, no one is sure whether reflux causes hiccups or the reverse. It doesn't matter to the patient as long as he or she is cured.

Constantine was the owner of a Greek restaurant who was referred to me by a surgeon in an effort to prevent an operation for chronic hiccups. Over three years he had been tried on every medication from Maalox to Prozac with no success. (The Prozac at least made him somewhat happier about his condition.) I placed Constantine on a high dose of Prilosec for two weeks, and his hiccups disappeared. He never required surgery.

Other parts of the body related to the nose and throat may be affected by acid reflux. I have already mentioned tooth decay (usually an erosion of the back of the teeth) and bad breath after consuming mints. Acid reflux sufferers may also get an acid taste in the mouth and increased salivation. None of these symptoms should surprise you when you consider the closeness of the affected organs. The stomach, lungs, esophagus, and voice box all are located within a few inches of one another (see figure 2). If you recall that stomach juice is almost as corrosive as the acid in your car battery (which is housed in a lead container), it shouldn't be difficult to understand how much injury gastric juice can cause if it escapes the stomach.

As with heartburn, human beings have attempted to deal with throat problems with humor. When we smile at the thought of the young lover trying to croak out a marriage proposal, the politician rasping through a windy speech, the speaker approaching the podium with a lump in her throat, we are minimizing these difficulties. Because no verifiable cause was known to account for all these symptoms, sufferers were branded hypochondriacs and hysterics, so we laughed helplessly or perhaps hung our heads in despair.

It is reassuring that we are now uncovering scientific proof that many of our ear, nose, and throat problems are not a product of mental delusion. It is further encouraging that hoarseness, loss of voice, and other related ills can be diagnosed and in many cases successfully treated.

8

CHEST PAIN

Heart Attack or Heartburn?

> Many patients die of a heart attack because they deny their chest pain and do not get help quickly enough. The first two hours are the most important. It is critical that patients arrive rapidly in a setting where trained doctors and nurses can prescribe lifesaving treatments.
> *—Elliott M. Antman, M.D., director, Levine Cardiac Unit, Brigham and Women's Hospital, Boston*

I recall the incident vividly. A woman in her late fifties rushed into a crowded emergency room with her husband. She had had a previous history of a heart attack and was now experiencing crushing chest pain. When the couple arrived, they feared that the woman would at best be hospitalized for days or at worst die from a second, lethal attack.

"Chest pain" is an automatic ticket past the long lines of sick, huddled masses waiting nervously in somber clumps on the vinyl chairs and couches of big-city emergency rooms. If you are having a heart attack, you speed right by because a few seconds determine whether you will live or die.

The woman was hurried to a treatment room, quickly surrounded by physicians and nurses feeling for a pulse, listening to her lungs, shining lights in the pupils of her eyes, and attaching her to an EKG machine to measure heart functioning. The woman's pain begin to intensify, and her body squirmed with tension. An increasingly elevated blood pressure reading indicated that her condition was worsening. An orderly wheeled in a "crash cart" with special equipment to reactivate her heart in case it slowed to a dangerously low rate or stopped.

Suddenly the patient's face contorted, and she let out a loud belch. Much to the astonishment and delight of staff and husband, the expiration of trapped gas from the woman's digestive system immediately ended both the patient's chest pain and the doctors' anxiety. I recall the scene so vividly because my eleven-year-old son, Matt, happened to race into the living room and change the television show I was watching with the remote control. By the time I got *ER* back on, the medical emergency was over.

In the usual television manner, a major public health problem affecting six hundred thousand new patients a year was dramatized and *solved* in about two minutes. The depiction of a patient with what doctors call noncardiac (not heart-related) chest pain was correct. Unfortunately, while the fictional solution was dramatic and funny, the real problem almost always takes a lot longer to solve.

Several new studies of patients who enter an emergency room with noncardiac chest pain indicate that many are not properly diagnosed for one *year* after the initial hospital admission. As a result, they are given the wrong therapy as well as needless tests, and they remain anxious and depressed. Again and again they race to emergency rooms and are sometimes hospitalized. It does not have to happen.

The emergency room is indeed a place where medical decisions are instantly made. As a medical resident in a very busy Philadelphia hospital I spent many sleepless hours working around the clock to treat patients and save lives. Few patients create so much tension in the ER as one who enters with a possible heart attack. The first rule for any such person is to find out how serious his or her condition is and to do so immediately.

Of the million or more patients who enter the hospital with crushing chest pain, about *half* have heartburn or reflux disease. We estimate this by the fact that many patients are simply discharged from the hospital once tests show their heart function is normal. Annually 600,000 undergo a procedure, cardiac catheterization, to determine whether the arteries to the heart itself are blocked. As surprising as it might seem, 180,000 of these people have no significant blockages at all. Their arteries are normal. (It is certainly possible that the woman depicted in the fictional *ER* would have had this procedure had she not conveniently belched.)

What really happens to people with noncardiac chest pain? In one survey they were found on average to receive 1.2 prescription medications per month, to visit a physician 2.2 times per year, and to have been hospitalized approximately once a year for further heart disease evaluation. How much does this cost? At least $750 million a year.

So overwhelming is this problem that several medical centers are starting programs to call a gastroenterologist *immediately* once a heart attack has been ruled out. If a diagnosis of heartburn, rather than heart disease, can be quickly made, the disease can be treated and corrected in a few weeks. Maybe not as fast as in *ER*, but a lot faster than it is now.

Separating heart attack from heartburn can be one of the most difficult diagnostic problems a physician faces. Doctors have long confused the two conditions, and indeed, they have similar names. The Latin name for the area of the stomach just below the esophagus is the *cardia*. Patients with heartburn are said to have cardialgia. Patients with heart disease are said to have cardiac illness.

Studies have established that neither skilled gastroenterologists nor cardiologists can successfully tell what kind of chest pain a patient has on the basis of a patient history alone. In other words, a patient may never have had heartburn and enter an emergency room with a heart attack or heartburn. The symptoms are exactly the same.

What exactly is a heart attack and what is noncardiac chest pain?

When a patient is having a heart attack, the heart muscle starts to die. Because the heart is itself a muscle that pumps blood throughout the body, the death of the heart muscle means the patient is in danger of severe illness or death. Many people do not report chest pain because they die before getting medical help. Within the heart is a regulator that is responsible for the automatic beating of the heart. If this regulator is destroyed by the death of the heart muscle, the patient's heart malfunctions and the patient dies quickly.

The heart muscle dies because it is cut off from the supply of life-sustaining blood containing oxygen and nutrients. The arteries delivering this nourishment become blocked by a blood clot (or any other substance), and the heart muscle soon perishes.

Doctors formerly believed that once a heart attack began, it could not be reversed. However, we now know that the process can be reversed either by drugs that dissolve blood clots or by insertion of a balloon into the artery. (The balloon is placed inside the blocked artery and inflated, crushing the obstructing clot and opening the passageway.) Both the drug and balloon therapy (known as angioplasty) quickly allow blood to flow again through the artery and prevent further damage. The faster the treatment, the less likelihood of physical harm or death to the patient. Hence, the scene of high drama in *ER*.

The chest pain from a heart attack occurs because the lack of oxygen to the heart muscle sets off a number of chemical abnormalities. The abnormalities are warning signals that are transmitted to nerves in the shoulders, chest, and arms and can cause intense pain. What is astonishing about this heart attack pain is how similar it can be to that of heartburn—so similar, in fact, that an expert on this subject was personally misled into making an almost fatal mistake.

I am speaking about myself.

I have for many years had mild heartburn, which is easily controlled by antacids, Tagamet, or Zantac. Although, like many Americans, I could stand to lose a few pounds, I am in good physical condition. I run every day or ride an exercise bike in rainy or cold weather. Other than being a male over the age of forty and having to drive to and from work in Boston rush-hour traffic, I have no risk factors for the development of heart disease. I do not smoke and have low cholesterol and normal blood pressure.

So much for the good news.

The morning of January 14, 1994, was bitterly cold. I rode my exercise bike, took the kids to school, and had a seemingly normal day at work. That night I ate a light dinner of chicken and rice with a glass of juice, read a medical journal, and went to sleep.

I awoke at one-thirty in the morning with severe chest pain. My years of studying reflux disease made me *sure* this was heartburn, so I got out of bed, took two Mylanta tablets, and tried to go back to sleep. Relief did come after several minutes, but it did not last, and I continued to have chest pain on and off for the next three hours.

At five in the morning I awoke feeling as if a vise were tightening around my chest. I lay in bed for fifteen minutes in terrible pain, reviewing my symptoms as if I were an outside diagnostic consultant. . . . Fortunately my wife awakened, took a quick look at me, and made the instant and correct decision: "Mike, I'm calling the rescue squad."

As I was being rushed to the Brigham and Women's Hospital, a member of the rescue team shook his head as I related the night's events and my long delay getting help. "Typical doctor," I remember him saying. "You're lucky to be alive."

Arriving at the Brigham, I felt like the character in *ER*. Except this time I was the patient clutching his chest and staring upward as a blur of figures rushed around me. The young cardiologist on call knew me and seemed more upset than I was. As if rehearsing for a canceled situation comedy, he actually blurted, "My *heart* goes out to you." I swear that I replied as a gastroenterologist, "I had the *gut* feeling you would say that."

There were a number of groans from nearby staff, some of whom knew me. "As long as he's still got a sense of humor, maybe we can keep him alive," said a doctor taping electrodes to my body.

It's strange how vividly you remember a critical situation. The emergency room banter made me think about how often I try to ease patients' fears with humor and how, faced with a day of medical disasters, I often use humor myself to keep the surrounding human suffering in perspective.

Within a few minutes I was engulfed by an expert team of cardiologists. The senior member of the group explained that he was going to insert a balloon into the artery that was blocked and get rid of the obstruction. "Fine," I croaked, "whatever you think is right."

"Why didn't you get here sooner?" he asked.

No sense lying on what might be your last morning on earth. "I thought I had heartburn."

"That figures," the cardiologist said. "Typical doctor."

Fortunately the angioplasty was successful, and I made a fast recovery, although I had much time to think about and research the difference in sensation between heart attack chest pain and heartburn chest pain. Surprisingly little is known. I asked an older, very distinguished colleague what differentiates the two ailments, and he replied, "Michael, if you ignore the chest pain caused by heart attack, you will surely die, and if you ignore the chest pain caused by heartburn, you will surely *want* to die."

I can personally attest to this fact.

Normally a person cannot feel his or her heart, but the muscle that drives the organ does have pain endings. When the heart is deprived of oxygen, a number of chemicals are released into the body. These chemicals activate the pain receptors in the heart and also travel along the nervous system to the upper chest, left arm and left shoulder, and neck. The reason pain moves along this path is that in the developing embryo in the mother's womb, the heart and arms evolve in the neck and share the same parts of the nerve system by which pain is transmitted.

The chest pain associated with GERD is also caused by the inability of the esophagus to deal with acid refluxing from the stomach. As with the other illnesses associated with reflux (such as asthma and hoarseness), acid is invading a sensitive portion of the esophagus that is damaged by this corrosive substance. Scientists do not know the precise location of this area within the esophagus, but they believe that when it is irritated, it causes the sensation of chest pain.

In any case, no one can tell the two types of chest pain apart without sophisticated electronic equipment. The reasons for the diagnostic difficulty go beyond those I have already described. They include the fact that both heart attack and heartburn are more likely to occur in people over the age of forty.

In addition, *both* illnesses may be present in many people. Reports indicate that one half the people with heart disease *also* have reflux disease. It is possible, therefore, that a patient coming into an emergency room has both heart disease and heartburn.

The personal histories of both kinds of patients may be similar. Patients with heart disease often complain of chest pain after exercise, but so do people with heartburn. The medical name for the condition of people with heart disease who experience chest pain is angina pectoris or angina. We test for angina by putting people on a treadmill and carefully monitoring their heart rate and symptoms as they walk and run in place. Heartburn patients frequently complain of similar feelings on the treadmill.

I used to tell my students that one of the key differences between heart disease and heartburn was that the latter was more likely to occur in the middle of the night. Obviously I don't teach this idea anymore.

Modern physicians first thought that heartburn in the chest started because of abnormal contractions in the esophagus. In 1899 a doctor named Hamilton Osgood suggested that such patients should be given "nitrate of silver," now commonly known as nitroglycerin. Nitroglycerin is frequently given to patients with heart disease and relieves their symptoms. It may also relieve the symptoms of some heartburn patients with chest pain.

In the same decade Sir William Osler, of Johns Hopkins, maintained that emotions were the cause of the quivering esophagus. The condition was found in "hysterical patients and hypochondriacs . . . especially females of a marked neurotic habit and elderly men." You may recall that these same hysterics also had asthma, skin disease, and various stomach ailments. Later, in the movies of the silent era, "damsels in distress" generally clutched at their chests and—if things got bad enough—fainted into the arms of tall, handsome, able-bodied males.

Dr. Wilder Tileston, earlier identified as the first American physician to diagnose ulcers of the esophagus, stated in 1905 that one of the symptoms of this disease was chest pain so severe it required morphine to treat. Interestingly Tileston suggested that patients with ulcer of the esophagus also be treated with silver nitrate and bismuth.

Later in the century other researchers found links among heartburn, reflux disease, and chest pain, but the relationship was not scientifically tested until the 1950s, when experiments conclusively demonstrated the correlation between acid in the esophagus and chest pain. Even so, controversy remained.

When I was training in gastroenterology in the late 1970s and early 1980s, conventional medical wisdom was clearly on the side of those who believed that noncardiac chest pain was caused by abnormal contractions in the esophagus, not by acid. As a result, many patients with this complaint were given drugs that relieved what was termed esophageal spasm. The most popular of these medications are called calcium channel blockers, Procardia and Cardizem. It was later learned that these drugs actually make reflux *worse* by easing the upward passage of stomach contents.

Not until the mid-1980s did we have more evidence that chest pain could be related to acid reflux. The proof came only partly because of more advanced diagnostic equipment. Reflux disease associated with chest pain (like asthma and loss of voice) may not show up with the usual tests. In many cases the esophagus is normal, and there is nothing unusual on any form of X ray.

The simplest way to test if chest pain is caused by reflux disease is simply to eliminate stomach acid production by a few weeks of medication. Experiments first performed in the 1980s and 1990s showed that about 60 percent of patients given high doses of histamine blockers (Tagamet, Zantac, Axid, Pepcid) experienced relief of noncardiac chest pain symptoms, and even more patients (80 to 90 percent) got relief of noncardiac chest pain with Prilosec.

This finding is revolutionizing emergency room medicine, and it is my hope that the effects will be even more far-reaching.

It is particularly ironic to me, given my own history and my profession, that physicians have dwelled on a psychological origin of chest pain. Anyone who has ever felt the sensation of a vise around the chest feels terror. Those who experience this condition regularly are naturally prone to panic.

Many patients who see me for their chest pain have been taking drugs like Valium or Xanax. They are also taking Procardia or wearing nitroglycerine patches. Few actually have anything wrong with their hearts. They have been tested and retested. But they are still worried about a potentially fatal condition *that they do not have*. Of course they have anxiety!

While chest pain patients must first make sure they do not have heart disease, they must also find out if they have reflux disease. A great many do, and once serious heart disease is excluded, their best bet would be to see a gastroenterologist as soon as possible.

If a specialist is not available, talk to your family doctor. Some of the finest physicians are primary care doctors, and if they know you well, they may be able to help you as well as or better than the specialist.

A good family doctor can also direct you to a person like me if the need arises. That is how I first saw Jerry, a fifty-two-year-old Boston businessman. Jerry had a high-pressure job and was going through a stressful divorce. The night following a major sales banquet he awoke at two with severe chest pain, nausea, and sweating. This was not the first time it had happened. On other occasions antacids brought relief. But Jerry realized that *this* time was different. Unlike me, Jerry did not spend the next few hours trying to diagnose himself.

He immediately dialed 911 and asked for emergency help. Once in the hospital, he was given a full evaluation, including blood tests, chest X rays, and an EKG. His heart function was normal, and his arteries were clear. However, when he related his medical history to the emergency room staff, he said that he "constantly" suffered from heartburn. "That's normal, isn't it?" Jerry said. "Everybody in my business has it."

No, it's not normal, and the fact that Jerry had chest pain made him forget his heartburn. I treated Jerry with Prilosec twice a day, and he has had no further attacks of either chest pain or heartburn.

What are my overall recommendations?

First, anyone with chest pain needs an evaluation for heart disease. Anyone with severe chest pain needs immediate medical attention.

Mild chest pain caused by reflux may occasionally be relieved with antacids. But don't rely on them. If you're constantly taking antacids for more than two weeks, you are suffering needlessly. If you have been to an emergency room, clinic, or even your own doctor and have not received a clear diagnosis for your condition, see a gastroenterologist or cardiologist.

If you have noncardiac chest pain and are taking medications that do not give you relief, you should also see a specialist—quickly. (But don't stop taking medication unless directed by a physician to do so.)

Some people with chest pain find relief with Tagamet or Zantac, but a high-dose course of Prilosec for a few weeks will help make it possible for your doctor to know if your chest pain is related to acid reflux. If reflux is the cause, you should get rapid symptom relief. You will also save yourself the needless expense and anxiety of hospital emergency room visits.

My final word on this subject is that the ER is a good place for television programs, an exhausting place for physicians to practice medicine, and a tremendous help for those with a medical crisis. But I do not care to go back as a patient; one time was enough.

9

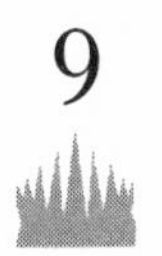

THE FUTURE

> The concept that disease results from failure to behave according to natural laws accounts in part for the fact that illness is more often accompanied by a sense of guilt than are other misfortunes. Even if he cannot identify his errors, the patient is likely to experience something akin to shame arising from a subconscious sense of responsibility for his fate.
>
> —*Dr. René Dubos,* Mirage of Health, Utopias, Progress, and Biological Change, *1959*

The eating and enjoyment of food are a powerful force in our lives from the earliest breath. Watch an infant crying for milk, a child screaming for food, an entire civilization migrating for more sustenance. Eating governs our religions, our festivals, our celebrations, our customs.

The makers of antacid commercials have an uncommon grasp of this elemental urge. People offer one another Tums tablets as if it were an act of faith: "Here, try one of these; it will save your soul." With one swig from an antacid bottle, a party bursts to life, passion ignites, the good times roll.

Unfortunately life is more complicated than a thirty-second television commercial, and the warnings and limitations about antacids flash by too quickly to see.

They work for only short periods of time, and they can neutralize only a limited amount of acid.

Regardless, the advertisements are a testimony to the extraordinary lengths people will go to avoid modifying a lifestyle that may cause acid reflux but increase pleasure. I believe it is my obligation as a physician to counsel patients about foods and actions that may jeopardize their health, but the reaction I get is usually the same. "Do you think I don't know about the dangers of drinking or smoking? Do you think I haven't *tried* a hundred times to lose weight? Take it easy? Why don't *you* try working for my boss? Do you want to take care of *my* three teenagers?" Then the inevitable request: "I came to you because I want medication."

If there is one philosophy my patients seem to express most frequently it is "Eat, drink and be merry, for tomorrow . . ." Indeed, following all the rules of good lifestyle does not guarantee health or anything else, for that matter—a not-so-well-kept secret that doctors well know. For whether they work in big-city hospitals or rural clinics, they see a constant torrent of random suffering. People get ill and die for no reason that we can figure out.

I had a great deal of time to meditate about this after I had my heart attack. My lifestyle was moderate, and I had no recognizable risk factors. I had received preventive medical checkups that left no doubt that I was in excellent health. Nonetheless . . .

One of the challenges of medicine is to develop more effective devices and tests with which bodily malfunctions can be quickly and precisely identified. Perhaps a simple test in the near future will be able to pinpoint the cause of heart attacks and help prevent them from occurring. We can now visualize with CT and MRI scans diseases that a few decades ago were thickly shrouded. In 1994 a group of researchers actually scanned and photographed the changes taking place inside the brain during a migraine headache. The results are already being analyzed to provide scientists with more clues to the origins and potential cures for this illness.

Certainly we need better diagnostic tools and methods to screen patients for acid reflux, especially where there is no obvious physical damage. Other silent diseases can quickly and easily be detected. For example, if a patient has high blood pressure (a disorder with no symptoms), a physician can uncover the condition with a painless test that takes less than a minute. Similarly, high cholesterol can be documented with a blood test and analyzer in a few minutes. However, acid reflux of many kinds can elude even expensive and complicated diagnostic procedures that take more than a day to perform.

This leaves us with perplexing questions: How can reflux patients have so much damage to their bodies but experience no pain or other symptoms? Conversely, how can patients have so much heartburn, chest, or asthmatic distress and no visible damage to vital organs or tissues?

One answer may lie in the subjective nature of pain itself, the fact that some people have higher thresholds of pain than others. Each human being has a unique ability to respond to stimuli from both external and internal sources. One person may be able to sleep soundly through a terrific thunderstorm, while another may be awakened by the drip of water in the next room. Football players make spectacular runs with broken arms, while armchair athletes with slight bruises groan at the thought of walking to the kitchen for more popcorn.

A personal example: I awaken with one chirp of my beeper or one ring of the phone in the middle of the night, slam doors getting dressed, drive to the hospital—and never awaken my wife. However, one peep from a baby is enough not only to wake my wife but to get her moving at full speed.

There's something ironic too. As we have learned more about the wide variety of illnesses for which acid reflux is responsible, our diagnostic tests have become less and less reliable. When reflux was simply thought of as the main cause of heartburn and esophagitis, the endoscope—which actually lets us look at the gullet—served us well. But the endoscope does not tell us much about asthma, hoarseness, or noncardiac chest pain. It does not even always let us "confirm" severe heartburn.

Thinking about it, I wonder how little we physicians have changed from our eighteenth-century predecessors who, unable to find anything wrong with their wheezing, coughing, indigestion-ridden patients, ascribed their ailments to "nervous liquors—hysteria—hypochondria."

We pay dearly for our lack of understanding, in terms of both the billions of dollars spent to treat and diagnose acid reflux and the continued suffering from which no one is immune. Political leaders ail along with the Boston cop, the midwestern church worker, and the Los Angeles lawyer. I have carefully laid out the steps to treat this malady and pointed out that many people with mild and occasional forms of acid reflux can be successfully treated with antacids. But as I also pointed out, antacids have certain limitations.

Because of this fact, in the late 1980s I began working on a new approach for people with mild, episodic heartburn: a combination of an antacid with an H2 blocker drug like Tagamet or Zantac. The antacid provides rapid relief from pain because the acid that has been created is immediately neutralized. At the same time the patient's acid production is turned off for hours by the H2 blocker.

This combination means that you won't have to keep taking antacids throughout the day to relieve your heartburn. By the time your first antacid tablet or liquid has lost its power, the H2 blocker will have reduced the production of acid that is the source of the problem.

Why did it take so long to come up with this idea? An important study published in the early 1980s demonstrated that antacids hindered the absorption of Tagamet and other H2 blockers into the bloodstream, thereby reducing their effectiveness. On the basis of this research and because of warnings of this interaction in various therapy guides used by doctors such as the *Physicians' Desk Reference* (*PDR*), many clinicians advise their heartburn patients *not* to use antacids when taking their H2 blockers.

Because the H2 blockers may take up to an hour or more to work, many patients have become dissatisfied with them. Who wants to wait for the distress of heartburn to go away? No one. Accustomed to the quick relief that antacids provide, patients expect their new drug to work the same way. It doesn't do that.

In my own studies I found that while antacids might have a slight impact on the potency of H2 blockers, this effect has little relation to how my patients actually *feel*. Patients on H2 blockers and antacids get just as lasting and effective relief as do those with H2 blockers alone.

On July 20, 1993, I obtained a patent from the United States Patent Office for treating mild episodic heartburn with a combination of H2 blocker and antacid. A carefully formulated medication combining these drugs is likely to be on the market within a few years. The product will probably be available to consumers without prescription and will provide both immediate (antacid) and sustained (H2 blocker) relief.

Meantime, you can try this form of therapy if you wish. Discuss the combination drug approach with your doctor. See if you can work out a schedule for taking your antacid and H2 blocker medications at the same time.

About one half to two thirds of heartburn patients who seek medical attention are helped by the prescription-strength doses of H2 blocker drugs. The other have a number of choices. If they are taking this type of medication only once a day, they can talk to their health providers about changing the strength and frequency of the dose.

Another option is to take a drug that aids the digestive process, Propulsid. Like the H2 blockers, Propulsid is a short-acting drug and needs to be taken two to four times a day. Some doctors prescribe a combination of H2 blockers and Propulsid. In patients with moderate to severe heartburn, this will require them to take from four to eight tablets a day.

The other alternative is to take one Prilosec capsule in the morning before breakfast. This will eliminate the problem of heartburn in more than 90 percent of patients. Some patients may have to take Prilosec twice a day for more severe forms of the illness.

A prime consideration today is cost. One Prilosec tablet is less expensive than four prescription-strength Tagamet tablets (the least expensive H2 blocker) and much less expensive than taking the combination of

Tagamet and Propulsid. Prilosec may also help reduce both the expense and the difficulty of making a diagnosis. As I've pointed out, patients who have acid reflux related to lung illness, hoarseness, loss of voice, and chest pain will not find the diagnostic process easy. An endoscopy will indicate problems in only about 25 percent of patients with reflux-related chest pain. (That may be one of the reasons why patients with this problem go so long without receiving proper medical care.) Endoscopy is not an effective tool for evaluating reflux-related lung disease or voice problems.

The best test for these conditions is a twenty-four-hour pH probe. The problem is that while this procedure is not nearly as bad as it sounds, about 5 percent of patients cannot tolerate it at all. Moreover, 15 percent alter their lifestyle (eat and drink less, change exercise habits) during the performance of the test in such a way that the results are meaningless.

The most practical option is to take a high-dose course (two capsules a day) of Prilosec for a few weeks and carefully note—and inform your physician—what changes occur. Asthmatics should notice a decrease in the need for inhalers and a better lung function. Those with chest pain should notice a decrease in attacks and a lessening of symptoms. (There is no "objective" way of measuring the decrease in noncardiac chest pain.) Patients with hoarseness should have a slow and steady improvement in the strength of their voices and the sound quality. The distress associated with speaking or swallowing should start disappearing.

Your doctor may be able to see a decrease in the swelling or inflammation around your vocal cords.

Not every patient will respond. I do not want to leave the impression that each person with one of these debilitating illnesses will get better. What I am saying is that antireflux treatment may provide hope to many who have not responded to any other therapy.

If high doses of Prilosec do not work, you may need surgery for your condition. Years ago this was the only alternative for people with severe reflux disease. Initially the surgical procedure involved repair of a hiatal hernia. But this operation did not prove effective because the hiatal hernia was not the primary cause of acid reflux. In the 1960s surgeons found a way to "tighten" the valve between the esophagus and the stomach by actually tying a wrap around it. This prevented acid and food from refluxing and doing damage to the esophagus. However, the success rate with this operation depends very much on the skill of the surgeon. I personally would consider it only with patients who have no other recourse.

Since the late 1980s researchers have developed a technique to perform the same basic antireflux procedure with a device known as a laparoscope. This instrument consists of a long tube with a video chip on the end that allows a surgeon to enter the body through a small hole. Tools are inserted into an area near the esophagus, and the surgeon can operate by watching a video screen.

This operation is becoming increasingly popular, and preliminary results are promising. But like the conventional procedure, it does not always work and has a number of side effects. The wrapping that tightens the valve and prevents reflux from occurring does not always stay in place. In addition, at least 10 to 15 percent of patients are left feeling uncomfortable and bloated.

We do not know at this time whether medication or surgery is more successful for severe reflux disease patients. The only careful study of this subject was performed before the availability of Prilosec and laparoscopic surgery. Of course, you, the patient, must make the final decision. If you are satisfied with your medication, feeling good and functioning normally, you do not need a study to tell you about the merits of surgery. On the other hand, if you have not responded to *any* medication, you may be left with no choice.

I base my own advice for patients on such factors as personal and family history, type and severity of reflux disease, lifestyle, and age. For example, some patients simply don't tolerate medication well and do not wish to take it for the rest of their lives. Other patients may have had poor responses to surgery or have health problems that would make an operation too risky.

Until we have more scientific research, the decision of which therapeutic course to take will have to be a personal one between patient and physician. Fortunately the overwhelming majority of acid reflux sufferers will respond quickly and almost completely to medication and never have to face this decision.

Few absolutes exist in medicine, but as I hope this book has made clear, recent advances against acid reflux have made it readily treatable. What many sufferers need most is recognition of their problem, proper medical attention, and the support of family, friends, and health providers. The government too needs to start taking a more active role, in both supporting research and expanding educational efforts.

Perhaps most important, our attitudes need to change. I hope never again to see patients with severe disease who have delayed treatment because they were embarrassed or feared ridicule.

In a society ever more conscious of medical costs, we cannot afford to waste billions of dollars because of unneeded visits to emergency rooms, hospital stays, loss of work, and outdated medication. Our lives are too precious to have them consumed with pain, and our health too important to jeopardize by ignorance, shame, and fear. If the knowledge in this book is given voice, the once-silent illness will be well on its way to being conquered.

APPENDIX

Lifestyle Modification in the Treatment of Acid Reflux

Physical Maneuvers

Avoid bending at the waist; bend at the knees.
Elevate the head of your bed with three- to six-inch blocks; or purchase a firm rubber wedge, such as the Bedge (800-525-4820).
Avoid tight-fitting garments.
Lose extra weight.

Foods to Avoid

Orange and other citrus juices and fruits
Coffee, including decaffeinated
Other caffeinated beverages, such as cola and tea
Spicy tomato juice
Fatty foods, including milk and other dairy products

Chocolate
Peppermint
Any food that specifically bothers *you*

Drugs to Avoid, if Possible
(Always Consult Your Physician First)

Long-acting nitroglycerin preparations
(Isordil, sorbitrate, isosorbide dinitrate, others)
Calcium channel blockers
(Calan, Procardia, Cardizem, others)
Tricyclic antidepressants
(Elavil, Tofranil, Pamelor, others)*
Weak blockers of acid production
(Pro-Banthāne, Bentyl, Valpin, others)
Drugs used to treat asthma
(Theo-Dur, Proventil tablets/elixir, Alupent tablets/elixir, many others)

Deleterious Chemicals

Tobacco use in general, but especially cigarette smoking
Alcoholic beverages

Beneficial Food Substances

Chewing gum
Sucking candy

*Newer antidepressants (Prozac, Paxil, Zoloft) generally do not cause heartburn.

GLOSSARY

Acid-neutralizing capacity (ANC)—the measure of the capacity of an antacid to neutralize stomach acid.

Acid pump inhibitor—a drug that blocks the ability of the stomach to produce acid; presently two are in use: Prilosec (omeprazole) and Prevacid (lansoprazole).

Acid (or reflux) laryngitis—injury to the voice box produced by the reflux of acid from the stomach and through the entire length of the esophagus.

Acid pump—a part of the stomach where acid is actually produced and "pumped" out for use.

Angina (pectoris)—chest pain caused by blockage of arteries leading to the heart itself. The precise mechanisms leading to pain are unknown.

Angioplasty—procedure in which a balloon is placed in

a blocked artery and inflated, crushing an obstructing clot and opening the artery.

Antacid—a drug that neutralizes acid present within the stomach. Generally composed of aluminum hydroxide and/or magnesium hydroxide, sodium bicarbonate, or calcium carbonate.

Asthma—a disease of the air passages characterized by difficulty in pulling air into and, to a greater extent, out of the lungs.

Axid (nizatidine)—an H2 blocker.

Barrett's esophagus—the transformation of the lining of the esophagus to a lining resembling that seen in the stomach. It can progress to a form of esophageal cancer. Produced by long-standing reflux of acid from the stomach into the esophagus and often viewed as a means of protection against the corrosive properties of acid. See also METAPLASIA.

Bedge—a firm foam wedge used to elevate the entire thorax that is used in lieu of elevating the head of the bed with blocks (similar devices are also available).

Bronchodilator—oral or inhaled drug that relaxes the airways, allowing easier movement of air into and out of the lungs.

Carafate (sucralfate)—a drug that coats the lining of the digestive tract; effective in healing ulcers of the stomach and duodenum.

Cardiac—referring to the heart.

Cardiac catheterization—a test performed on patients with chest pain to determine whether the pain is due to blocked arteries to the heart; also done in patients with structural abnormalities of the heart.

Duodenum—the first portion of twenty-five to thirty feet of small intestine. Located immediately beyond the stomach, it is the most common site of "peptic ulcers."

Endoscopy—a medical test in which a long, flexible tube is inserted through the mouth into the esophagus, stomach, and upper small intestine. The use of special lenses and fiberoptics or a video chip allows the physician to view the lining of the digestive tract and to obtain samples of the lining (biopsy).

Esophagitis (or peptic esophagitis)—inflammation of the lining of the esophagus most commonly caused by prolonged contact with stomach acid. It can range in severity from redness of the lining to severe ulceration and scarring.

Esophagus—the "food pipe" (or gullet) leading from the mouth and throat into the stomach.

Gastroenterologist—a physician (internist) who specializes in treating diseases of the digestive tract, including disorders of the esophagus, stomach, small intestine, colon (large intestine), liver, gallbladder, and pancreas.

Gastroesophageal reflux disease (GERD)—a disorder characterized by the reverse flow (reflux) of acid and other stomach contents from the stomach (gastro) back into the esophagus or food pipe (esophageal). See also GERD.

Gaviscon—a drug that contains alginic acid, a chemical that creates a foam barrier between the stomach and esophagus, thereby preventing acid reflux.

GERD—divided into erosive and nonerosive GERD depending on the presence or absence of acid-induced damage to the lining of the esophagus. See also GASTROESOPHAGEAL REFLUX DISEASE.

Globus sensation—the feeling of a lump in the back of the throat, possibly caused by acid reflux.

Heart attack—death of heart muscle because of blockage of arteries leading to the heart itself. The muscle does not receive oxygen and nutrients, leading first to reversible and later to irreversible damage.

Heartburn—a burning sensation that occurs beneath the breastbone and often radiates to the neck and shoulders as the result of the reverse flow (reflux) of acid from the stomach into the esophagus.

Hiatus (or hiatal) hernia—the abnormal protrusion of the stomach through the diaphragm and into the chest. Although uncommonly the cause of any symptoms, it may be associated with the reflux of acid into the esophagus.

H2 blocker or antagonist—a drug that diminishes the ability of histamine to stimulate the stomach to produce acid. Four are now in use: Tagamet (cimetidine), Zantac (ranitidine), Pepcid (famotidine), and Axid (nizatidine).

Laparoscope—instrument consisting of a long tube with a video chip on the end that is inserted by a surgeon into the body through a small hole. Tools are inserted through other small holes, and the surgeon operates by observing on a video monitor.

Larynx—the voice box at the opening to the lungs. It produces the sounds we use in everyday speech.

Metaplasia—the transformation of one type of body tissue to another by a process that can generally be regarded as a protective mechanism. Unfortunately metaplasia can also transform further into cancer. See also BARRETT'S ESOPHAGUS.

Pepcid (famotidine)—an H2 blocker.

Peptic ulcer—an open sore anywhere in the digestive tract produced by the corrosive effects of two chemicals, acid and pepsin (hence "peptic" ulcer). It most commonly occurs in the first portion of the small intestine, the duodenum, and the lower portion of the stomach, but it can also occur in the esophagus in more severe cases of GERD.

pH—a measure of the concentration of acid. The lower the pH, the greater the amount of acid, and vice versa.

pH probe—a thin, flexible tube and sensor that measure the amount of acid present in the esophagus over a period of time (usually twenty-four hours). It is used to determine whether symptoms like hoarseness, asthma, or chest pain are due to acid reflux.

Placebo—inactive sugar pill used for comparison when testing the effectiveness and safety of a new drug.

Prevacid (lansoprazole)—a blocker of the acid pump.

Prilosec (omeprazole)—a blocker of the acid pump.

Propulsid (cisapride)—a drug that improves digestion by moving food more rapidly through the digestive tract. Useful in GERD by tightening the sphincter between the stomach and esophagus and by hastening the clearance of refluxed food back into the stomach.

Reflux ("backflow")—the reverse flow of acid from the stomach to the esophagus.

Reglan (metoclopramide)—a drug that improves digestion by moving food more rapidly through the digestive tract. Somewhat useful in GERD by tightening the sphincter between the stomach and esophagus and by hastening the clearance of refluxed acid back into the stomach. Its use is limited by frequent side effects.

Simethicone—an inert ingredient often included in antacid formulations that breaks up gas bubbles in the stomach.

Sippy diet—bland diet consisting of hourly antacids alternating with milk. Named after the twentieth-century physician Dr. Bertram Sippy.

Sphincter (lower esophageal)—a protective barrier or valve between the esophagus and stomach that can be regarded as a one-way swinging door intended to allow food into the stomach. *Inappropriate* relaxation of this barrier allows acid to reflux into the esophagus.

Tagamet (cimetidine)—an H2 blocker.

Wheezing—high-pitched breath sounds characteristic of asthma and signifying difficulty in pulling air into and, to a greater extent, out of the lungs.

Zantac (ranitidine)—an H2 blocker.

Zollinger-Ellison syndrome—a disease characterized by enormous acid output by the stomach and ulcers of the esophagus, stomach, and duodenum.

INDEX